a Fighting
Chance

How to Win The War Against Bacteria, Viruses & Mold With Silver

Dr. Gordon Pedersen

CONTENTS

SECTION I
A FIGHTING CHANCE 5

SECTION II
THE SILVER SOLUTION 11

SECTION III
BACTERIA, VIRUSES AND MOLD 19

SECTION IV
WOMEN HAVE DISTINCT HEALTH CONCERNS............ 23

SECTION V
THE ESSENCE OF GOOD HEALTH 25

SECTION VI
GENERAL USES FOR BODY SYSTEMS......................... 39

SECTION VII
SILVER USES A-Z 44

SILVER SOL GEL USES 139

SECTION I

A FIGHTING CHANCE

It's no secret that pathogens such as viruses, bacteria and fungi can inflict terrible damage in the human body. Dozens of diseases—ranging from the common cold and dysentery to meningitis and pneumonia—are caused by infectious pathogens.

These diseases are all around us. We come in contact with countless bacteria everywhere we go. Bacteria are in restaurants, public restrooms, schools, airplanes—all spread by touch or passed through the air. Disease can even result from our own habits, like inadequate sleep or too much stress.

Currently, disease is winning the battle. Each year, we suffer from colds and the flu. Likewise, strep throat, sinus infections, and stomachaches attack our health.

Fortunately, a simple, safe, and effective solution exists. For decades, silver products have been marketed as medicinal agents for use primarily as disinfectants. In fact, patents on silver products have existed since the early 1920s. However, earlier versions of silver—called "colloidal silver"—had to be used in large amounts to be effective.

Currently, a new and vastly improved type of silver has been developed that is non-toxic and extremely effective against a wide range of bacteria, viruses, fungi, mold and other pathogens. This Silver Solution—called simply Silver Sol—is available as both a liquid and a gel.

Because we are faced with more diseases than ever before, we need a better solution than ever before. This book will outline some of the health threats facing our modern society and what we can do to have a fighting chance in this battle.

Antibiotics Provide Little or No Protection

We used to be confident that antibiotics would help us fight off disease. This is no longer true—the antibiotic era is drawing to a close. Pathogens are becoming increasingly dangerous and resistant strains are causing deadly outbreaks in hospitals, nursing homes, schools, and restaurants. Antibiotics are failing to outsmart microbes. They are being misused, overused and becoming ineffective.

Antibiotics have served to make our diseases drug resistant. On any given day in America there are 30,000 MRSA (methicillin resistant staph aureus) infections. We have overused antibiotics, making them ineffective in killing pathogens that have become increasingly resistant.

In a similar example, the Centers for Disease Control (CDC) recently sent a written notice to American physicians alerting them that no antibiotics were to be used on ear infections because they only make the infectious agent more resistant.

With all traditional options available to doctors for treating pathogenic infections nearly exhausted, doctors are virtually helpless to treat serious, virulent strains that may strike.

There is a need for a product or therapy that destroys bacteria, viruses and fungi without making the pathogens become resistant to the therapy.

Epidemic Inevitabilities

A few years ago, I had an experience I will never forget. I was in Singapore on the day of the SARS virus outbreak. I watched the mass hysteria as people rushed to make preparations to isolate themselves from any public human contact in hopes of avoiding the virus.

Everyone headed first to the local stores. Within four or five hours, shelves once filled with plastic, duct tape, air filters, water filters, and immune-stimulating supplements were completely empty. Within 24 hours, it was impossible to buy anything that would deter a viral infection. People didn't want to leave their homes. They did all they could think of to prevent the contagious disease, going so far as to drape entire apartment buildings in plastic.

While riding on a commuter train, I saw two nurses in surgical scrubs with hospital name tags step into the train. Everyone rushed out of the car when they saw them, fearing the nurses would expose them to the SARS virus from the hospital.

I found myself in a very interesting situation. Should I leave immediately before the car doors closed or was I confident that there was no risk? In the next second, every possible emotion ran through my head. At first I was afraid, but then I decided it was silly to think health care professionals would be contagious. I then realized the SARS Virus originated in a Singapore Hospital and these two nurses were wearing tags from that very hospital.

I leaned forward to leave, but hesitated after making eye contact with one of the nurses. I didn't want to offend them, but when I thought about my family, I instinctively hustled out of the car with the others. Better to be safe than sorry, I thought.

In the next few minutes I laughed at myself for the anxiety I felt when everyone else ran from the nurses. I should have known better. After all, these were health care professionals and I'm sure they took all the precautions necessary to prevent contamination. I was wrong. I later learned that half of the SARS casualties from that outbreak were health care professionals from that Singapore Hospital. I shuddered to think of how close I was to disaster.

This experience showed me firsthand how people respond to an emergency. We instinctively become anxious, aggressive survivalists. Many government and hospital workers choose to take vacation and stay home, crippling government facilities. Food and supply prices skyrocket. Emergency efforts fall short. In the end, we are left to fend for ourselves and our families.

An outbreak of contagious disease can happen anywhere and the threat of bioterrorism is always at hand. But what can we do? Fortunately, there are simple, effective ways to protect ourselves from these inevitabilities.

Contagious Diseases: Your Country Will Not Be Able To Protect You

I wish I could say that my experience in Singapore was an isolated event—something that could never happen in the United States. Unfortunately, that is not the case. You must not assume that your country can protect you in the case of a contagious outbreak.

During the first few weeks of any contagious disease outbreak, government agencies will not have sufficient staff, beds, drugs, prevention products, or time to assist all of the potentially millions of people needing help. Food and medical supplies will become scarce. You will likely need to care for yourself for the first few weeks of an outbreak.

Though the U.S. government's Department of Homeland Security has made admirable progress, it has yet to complete a national plan for an influenza pandemic. The government is stockpiling influenza vaccines in the event of an influenza outbreak, but the drugs often expire after one year. This leaves hundreds of millions of dollars of governmental support thrown away each year. Supplies are being accumulated and communities put on notice to organize emergency programs, but they are not yet in place.

During the Hurricane Katrina crisis, many people had to wait weeks before receiving medical attention. Others died of starvation in their own homes. I thought of how important it is for any family to have primary prevention stored in the home and a 72-hour pack ready if there were an epidemic or natural disaster.

Bio-Terrorism:
It Will Happen Again

In addition to natural disasters, man-made disasters are becoming more of a concern. For thousands of years, terrorists have created new weapons—swords, knives, catapults, gunpowder, bombs, and even nuclear weapons. Terrorists are now attacking with biological weapons, using bacteria, viruses, mold and parasites.

During times of war, people are capable of anything. As we look back at history, we see that humans could not restrain themselves from using nuclear weapons, Agent Orange, and biological warfare in their selfish attempt to advance a political cause. It is during these times that terrorists will release their most horrible weapons.

Governments and terrorists have been at war throughout history. Terrorists want to do as much harm to as many people as possible. Governments try to protect their citizens without losing control of the political environment. Unfortunately in this battle, peacekeeping residents are often left to defend themselves.

We are always at risk of a terrorist attack and none of us will forget what happened in New York City on September 11, 2001. If you want to survive a future bioterrorist attack, you must learn to protect yourself against biological weapons including bacteria, viruses and mold.

A Vision of the Future:
Doctors and Drugs Will Not Protect You

When a pandemic occurs, it will be irrelevant whether it was created by natural circumstances, or by nefarious individuals. You will only have a limited time to prepare your family and home for its consequences. In the worst cases, you may only have two or three hours to prepare. Imagine what will happen at local and regional stores—food, supplies, and medicine will be gone within hours. Trucks, planes and all forms of public transportation could cease. Your radio, television, phone and Internet could be regulated for emergency use only. Schools, hospitals and other large community facilities may become shelters, but only the unprepared and exposed will go there, making them the prime locations for the spread of disease. Your air, water, and food supplies may be contaminated. Healthcare professionals will be exposed to the pandemic's victims first, and may either die early or isolate themselves in the hospitals where you will not have access to them. Those that are available will be so overwhelmed with patients that you may have to wait days to get help. In all likelihood, you'll be forced to deal with the pandemic's consequences with your own knowledge and preparation.

Nontraditional Tools

Superbugs are winning the battle against disease but we can win the war by looking at nontraditional methods of fighting the microbial threat. New therapeutic silver preparations offer a safe and effective means of fighting pathogens where antibiotics and other drugs fail.

Silver can protect us from epidemic outbreaks, contagious diseases, and even bio-terrorist attacks by defeating the root of these problems—bacteria, viruses, and mold.

Research on silver is broad and spans several decades. Reputable labs at the University of Georgia, Kansas State University, Penn State, Arizona State, University of Arizona, University of California at Davis, and Brigham Young University are among those that have completed research supporting silver's use in fighting microbial infection. And newly patented technology has only increased the efficiency and safety of Silver Solutions.

SECTION II

THE Silver SolUTION

The History of Silver

Throughout history, silver has been used across the world as both a medicine and a preservative. In fact, hundreds of years before scientists and doctors understood microbes and how they cause illness, colloidal metals—particularly silver—were known for their health benefits.

Ancient Greeks used silver vessels for water purification. American pioneers trekking westward used silver to keep their water safe and to prevent dysentery, colds, and flu. They also put silver dollars in their milk containers and wooden water casks to slow bacterial growth. Settlers in the Australian outback suspended silverware in their water tanks to prevent spoilage. Topical silver antiseptic solutions were used during World War II. Even the superstition of throwing silver coins into a well is based on the legend of the metal's healing properties.

The use of silver for purification purposes continues today. Silver water purification filters are used in Switzerland and by international airlines, and silver catheters are used in hospitals. More recently, NASA has used silver in their space shuttle water purification systems. Silver is also used in residential homes. Electrical ionization units designed for swimming pools help sanitize the water without the harsh effects of chlorine.

Medicinal silver compounds were first developed in the late 1800s, and widespread use was common prior to 1930. By 1940, approximately 48 different silver compounds were on the market for treating a variety of ailments. These were available in oral, injectable, and topical forms and carried such names as Albargin, Novargan, Proganol and Silvol.

Since 1973, silver has been shown to have topical activity against 22 bacterial species (643 isolates), including gram-positive and gram-negative bacteria. The potential of silver in treating pathogenic infection is so great that the New York City board of physicians gave its stamp of approval for its use as a homeopathic medicine.

From silverware to silver foil, from silver eye drops to colloids and ionics, our scientific understanding of silver in all its forms has advanced considerably. But the foundation remains the same—silver has the ability to interfere with microbial growth and proliferation without harming the human body.

Interest in silver has grown in recent years due to the emergence of antibiotic-resistant superbugs and the growing ineffectiveness of many antibiotics. More than 95 percent of staph bacteria are now resistant to penicillin, the mother of antibiotics. In the 1960s, methicillin replaced penicillin as the standard staph treatment. Today more than 60 percent of staph bacteria are resistant to methicillin (called MRSA strains). A recent report from the *Journal of the American Medical Association* (JAMA) stated public health authorities estimate MRSA strains are causing more deaths in the United States than AIDS. Silver preparations, however, do not have this same problem with bacterial resistance; even MRSA strains and avian flu respond to therapeutic silver preparations.

What is Silver Sol and How Does it Work?

Silver Sol, in essence, is simply silver particles dispersed in purified water. The term "Sol" is a chemical designation of a pure mineral permanently suspended in water where the mineral's charge is transferred to the entire body of water. Differences between preparations are plenty; however, the silver concentration and the size of the particles can vary greatly, as can the bioavailability of the silver and the effectiveness of the solution. There are also variances in the purity of the solution. Solutions made with metallic silver are tested to be more potent than other silver preparations, such as those made with ionic silver. You may have heard of colloidal silver and ionic silver. While these can be effective solutions, I prefer the new silver technology called Silver Sol, also called Silver Aquasol technology.

Silver Sol preparations are manufactured by a completely different method, that in my opinion produces a far superior result. Silver Sol technology uses 10,000 volts of alternating current (AC), while the old colloids use 110 volts of direct current (DC). This significant increase in power essentially supercharges the silver, which results in a solution that has a different atomic structure than the colloids and ionics. The common colloid is missing one electron in its outer shell, which is why it can remove an electron from the bacteria and destroy it.

In this way colloids and ionic silvers have been very successful in destroying bacterial infections. Silver Sol is an Ag 404; it is missing two electrons in its outer shell, which consequently gives it catalytic capabilities. This capability can be described as one electron destroying bacteria, viruses, and mold while the other electron is being recharged. This catalytic conversion allows the Silver Sol to first destroy then to instantaneously recharge and "kill" again and again—like a rapid-fire machine gun. The result is that Silver Sol can destroy thousands of times more pathogens than a simple colloid or ionic silver. This means that Silver Sol can be much more effective at a very safe concentration (5-20 parts per million), which can potentially be consumed every day.

These newer silver preparations rely on engineered nano-particle solutions with higher bioavailability, effectiveness and safety. Metallic silver gives off ultra-violet radiation in narrow wavelengths. These wavelengths are tested to destroy a wide range of pathogens. The narrow wavelength energy radiated from silver produces free radicals that damage their DNA beyond repair. Silver doesn't even need direct contact with the microbe to create this effect.

Simply put, Silver Solutions interfere with the energy sources of bacteria, viruses and other microbes. The process is a bit complicated, but basically the charge of silver replaces needed hydrogen atoms, and the result is that it blocks energy sources that microbes need. This reaction can happen within minutes of exposure.

Because silver affects such a basic mechanism of normal microbial function, it is effective against a broad range of pathogens. Even if DNA or RNA structure varies or the mode of attack varies, the basic structure of the pathogen is the same and can be addressed by silver's nontraditional mode of attack. While typical drugs or antibiotics are effective against six or seven microbes, silver preparations are effective against more than 500 different disease-causing pathogens without encouraging drug resistance and without side effects. And a little goes a long way.

The Benefits of Silver

- Broad-spectrum antimicrobial (some silvers have been shown in vitro to destroy bacteria, both forms of viruses, fungus and other significant diseases including the following: MRSA, SARS, malaria, anthrax poisoning, gram-negative bacteria, gram-positive bacteria, Hepatitis C, AIDS, and influenza
- Potent anti-inflammatory
- Non-toxic, even at high levels
- No side effects or contra-indications; safe for all individuals
- Doesn't encourage resistant microbial strains
- Has prophylactic potential in disease prevention
- Immune system enhancer
- Cost-effective
- Internal and topical usage
- Works synergistically with prescribed antibiotics
- More effective than traditional antibiotics and other drugs

Silver Solution vs. Suspension

When discussing silver preparations, it is important to note the difference between a suspension and a solution. Basically, the difference is in the fineness of particles dispersed. Although particles in a suspension can't be seen, they are still large enough to settle at the bottom of the container over time. But electrically charged ions in a solution will not settle after weeks, months or years. The ideal Silver Solution perfectly straddles the line between a solution and a suspension because it maintains its molecular identity without large particles settling. While too small particles do not have the correct reactivity, particles of the proper size are more readily absorbed and more catalytically effective at killing pathogens before they are excreted by the body.

Not All Silver is Equal

Not all silver is equally effective. Old silver products were often brown or yellow. They contained more silver but were far less effective, often requiring 50,000 to 300,000 ppm (parts per million) of silver to kill a harmful pathogen. The new Silver Solution is colorless, odorless, and exhibits only a faint metallic aftertaste. It can terminate entire colonies of harmful bacteria at concentrations of 5 ppm or less.

Likewise, not all new silver products are the same. One product on the market has been shown to inhibit the growth of *E. coli* at 1,500 ppm. Silver Sol has been shown to kill *E. coli* at a concentration of only 2.5 to 5.0 ppm. That is several hundred times more effective than the colloids or ionic silver preparations.

Silver Sol is also much more bio-available than other silver technologies on the market. That means more of the silver is readily absorbed and utilized in the body. Researchers at Brigham Young University tested many current silver products. These products were found to have bioavailabilities between 15 and 65 percent. Silver Sol was then tested. It was not only more effective against microbes in laboratory tests, its bioavailability exceeded 99 percent.

Silver's Attack Strategies: Chemical Structure/Contact

Silver Sol particles are tiny enough to be absorbed into a single red blood cell. Pure silver is supercharged and surrounded by a chemical shell that is missing two electrons (called ionic because it carries a charge). This means the tiny silver particle wants to attach to the thin cell walls of pathogens and remove one or two electrons. This leaves a hole in the cell membrane and kills the pathogen. Normal cells have thicker, more protective cell membranes that have a balanced charge, resulting in selective protection from the silver's oxide coating that kills bacteria on contact.

Resonance

There are healthy and unhealthy resonances. For example, imagine a vibrating back massager compared to the jolting frequency of a jackhammer. In a similar way, silver resonates at a frequency selectively destructive to pathogens. In fact, it has been measured to resonate at 890 to 910 terahertz. This is the same frequency at which germicidal ultraviolet light resonates. Imagine now tiny silver particles that are small enough to be absorbed into the red blood cells, and resonate at the perfect frequency to destroy bacteria, viruses, and yeast. These tiny "flashlights" circulate throughout every capillary in the body, disinfecting from the inside.

Magnetic Disruption of Viral DNA

A virus is constructed of a capsid that contains incomplete segments of DNA and RNA. These DNA segments carry a slight magnetic charge. There is a claw on the outside of the virus that attaches the virus to a healthy cell. Once the virus is attached to a healthy cell it can "inject" the incomplete DNA into the healthy cell, producing damage to the normal DNA and causing it to reproduce abnormally. This can cause viral diseases like influenza, hepatitis, and cervical cancer.

The new supercharged silver acts like a magnet that attracts the charged DNA particles. The DNA binds so tightly to the silver that it makes a chaotic tangle of incomplete genetic material that can never lengthen out, so it can never go through replication. This inactivates the virus, preventing replication of the disease. Normal cells have thicker, more protective cell membranes with a balanced charge, which protects them from the silver's magnetic attraction.

Cellular Communication

Most cells communicate through a sugar—or saccharide—coating. This coating lets the cell know friend from foe. Silver has a "friendly" saccharide coating that allows it to positively communicate with cells. This way, silver nano-particles can enter into an abnormal cell and attack pathogens before they have a chance to replicate.

What the Research Says

Research on silver is broad and spans several decades. Reputable labs at the University of Georgia, Kansas State University, Penn State, Arizona State University, University of Arizona, University of California at Davis, and Brigham Young University are among those that have completed research supporting silver's use in fighting microbial infection. For complete studies, see section 9.

An MD testimonial letter reported the effective use of silver in more than 50 cases involving patients with viral pneumonia, as well as those with ear infections, infectious fibromyalgia, Sjorgen's syndrome, rheumatic arthritis, systemic Candida, staph, gingivitis, Lyme disease, HIV, ringworm, psoriasis, genital herpes, and herpes zoster.

In another study testing the effect of silver on the growth rate of spirochete Borrelia burgdorferi (the cause of Lyme disease) it was found that even low concentrations (between 2 and 10 ppm) were enough to visibly inhibit the bacteria.

A study out of Brigham Young University (BYU) testing the effectiveness of silver preparations on a wide range of microbes found that silver was a broad-spectrum antimicrobial able to kill a large variety of pathogens. In fact, none of the pathogens tested survived silver exposure.

Another BYU study compared the effect of silver with five antibiotics on seven different pathogens: E. coli B, E aerogenes, E cloacae, S typhimunium, P aeruginosa, S gordonii, and S aureus. While silver was able to kill all bacteria tested, the antibiotics did not work equally well on all bacteria.

Although some antibiotics were effective on some of the bacteria tested, only silver had effective results on all seven. A study out of the University of California at Davis also found silver to be effective against the yeast S. cerevisiae variant montrachet. One dose of silver at a concentration of 15 ppm was an effective inhibitor. Candida albicans was also inhibited at silver concentrations of 10 ppm or less. This is significant because fungal infections are especially hard to treat and are often resistant to drug treatments.

Silver is also useful in water treatment. Its ability to kill waterborne pathogens was tested in 1999 at a Utah lab. Low-level Silver Solutions were used on untreated river water and a 10-ppm concentration was effective in killing all bacteria colonies in less than four minutes. Another study tested silver on 50 gallons of raw sewage containing 7,000 E. coli cells per milliliter. After three hours of being flushed with silver electrodes, the sewage was contamination free.

Research on silver as a treatment for hepatitis B is also promising. When compared with standard hepatitis treatment, which doesn't cure the disease but does slow its progress, silver offered 89 percent inhibition without side effects. Standard treatment has a mere 18 percent effectiveness and is accompanied by several side effects.

When doctors in Ghana used silver preparation to treat resistant strains of malaria, all 50 patients showed no sign of blood parasites after five days of treatment.

Study Highlights

- Silver preparations were effectively used by one doctor to treat more than 50 cases of viral pneumonia with great success.

- The growth rate of spirochete *Borrelia burgdorferi*, the cause of Lyme disease, was inhibited at even low concentrations of between 2 and 10 ppm according to another recent study.

- A study out of Brigham Young University found silver to be a broad-spectrum antimicrobial that inhibited or killed all pathogens tested.

- Silver Sol was more effective than 19 antibiotics in killing seven different bacteria.

SECTION III

Bacteria, Viruses, Mold

In general, one teaspoon of Silver Sol is taken orally in the morning and at night. This offers a degree of protection against the myriad diseases we are exposed to every day. Since the transfer of 70 percent of all contagious diseases happens by touching things with your hands, applying a Silver Sol gel to your hands just as frequently may prevent this disease transfer for up to 4 hours. Now, these two recommendations are only a starting point. Later in the book you will see literally hundreds of uses and benefits of both Silver Sol liquid and Silver Sol gel. Silver's amazing health benefits are based on its ability to destroy bacteria, viruses, molds, and fungi.

Bacteria

Bacteria are single-cell organisms that grow within or outside your body. Left uninhibited, bacteria can cause disease or death. Many of today's health problems result from bacteria. Pneumonia, one of the leading causes of death in America, comes from bacteria inside of the lungs.

Silver Sol will destroy bacteria in approximately six minutes. You will feel the effects within the first two hours of use and the benefits will continue as long as you use the product. Consumption of Silver Sol should also be combined with that of vitamins, minerals, essential fatty acids, amino acids, and antioxidants.

Viruses

A virus is a sub-microscopic infectious agent that is unable to grow or reproduce outside a host cell. We generally fight viruses by using antibiotics. However, antibiotics do not actually destroy the virus. For many viruses, such as influenza or the bird flu, there are virtually no beneficial drugs or treatment.

Silver Sol resonates at a frequency that can actually suppress and contain viral infections by interfering with the duplication and replication of viral infections. If you can stop a virus from duplicating in the first four hours of infection, you have a good chance of stopping the symptoms entirely.

When the herpes virus infects the skin, we call it a canker sore or cold sore. If you use Silver Sol within the first four hours of feeling the sore, it will not even erupt. However, if you don't get it in the early phases, viral infection will duplicate and become much more difficult to control. This is why regular preventive use is so important.

To fight viruses, Silver Sol can be taken internally as a liquid, used topically as a gel, or inhaled to combat sinus problems. You can expect a noticeable benefit within the first two hours and significant benefits within the first two days.

Mold and Fungus

Fungus and mold grow in warm, moist, and sugared areas such as the intestines or vagina. Taking the sugar out of your diet and using silver both topically and internally can treat this propensity. Take two teaspoons of silver three times a day and apply it topically one to four times a day, if needed. This dosage should be continued for at least two weeks longer than symptoms are present.

You can expect to see a benefit within the first 30 minutes. It will take at least ten minutes for the liquid to kill a fungal infection on the skin. Silver will work best when taken with complementary products such as probiotics, caprylic acid, anti yeast diets, essential fatty acids, and amino acids.

Silver can also be sprayed on household items. In about ten minutes it will kill the fungi, bacteria, or viruses on your table, food, clothes, phone, refrigerator, or toilet.

Who Can Use Silver?

Because adults and children have a very similar response to silver, it can be used from the age of six months old until the last day of your life. Because this product does not mutate or cause bacteria to mutate and become resistant, it can be safely used every day.

Expected Results

Silver can be used anywhere on your body, both topically and internally. In general, you can expect to feel the silver begin working within minutes.

When liquid silver comes in contact with a germ, it will destroy it in an average of six minutes. For example, gargling liquid or gel silver for six minutes will kill all of the bacteria in the back of a sore throat.

Though you will feel the benefits quickly, the effects continue over days, weeks and even months as obstacles are removed from the immune system. By destroying bacteria, viruses, and mold, silver allows the immune system to focus entirely on building, healing, and protecting the rest of the body. With pathogens out of the way, healing can occur much more quickly.

Though silver maintains the widest spectrum of killing activity of any of the substances currently known, it will not kill everything immediately.

Evaluating Your Progress

How do you know if silver is working for you? There are two ways. The first is a reduction of symptoms. For example, you'll know a Silver Sol foot soak is working by the reduction of fungal infection under the toenail. The same can be said of a sore throat or earache that goes into remediation when using silver.

The second way is to look at your overall feeling of wellness. If you are experiencing less illness and experiencing better quality of life, you can be confident that silver is helping you prevent disease. Less disease means more opportunity for an active lifestyle and more time to spend with family and friends.

SECTION IV

Women Have Distinct Health Concerns

Women and men have many of the same health problems, but they can affect women differently. For example, women may have different symptoms of heart disease. Some diseases or conditions are more common in women, such as osteoarthritis, obesity and depression. And some conditions are unique to women—vaginal problems, menopause, etc. This book focuses on women's health concerns that result from bacteria, viruses or fungus, and the best way to treat those diseases.

On any given day about one in four women will suffer from some kind of vaginal problem, whether it be yeast infection, staph infection or human papillomavirus. These problems can range from irritating to life threatening. The vaginal cavity is a warm, moist cavity, making it the ideal place for the growth of bacteria, yeast and viruses. Problems can result from poor hygiene, contamination, hormonal issues or genetics. The most common vaginal problems are bacterial vaginosis and yeast infections. Disorders of the vaginal cavity are difficult to identify because the problems are not visible and a woman often doesn't know of the problem until symptoms manifest themselves. Pain, itchiness, redness, swelling, cramps, or abnormal bleeding are often the first signs of a problem. All of these symptoms respond to vaginal cleansing, both as a preventive measure and as treatment.

Solving the Problem with Silver Sol

The battle against illness and disease is ongoing. Women are constantly fighting infections of all types. Fortunately, a simple, safe, and effective solution exists. For decades, silver products have been marketed as medicinal agents for use primarily as disinfectants. Currently, a new and vastly improved type of silver has been developed that is non-toxic and extremely effective against a wide range of bacteria, viruses, fungus, mold and other pathogens. This silver solution—called simply Silver Sol—could be the instrument used by women everywhere to win the war against disease.

The fact that silver is antibacterial, antiviral and antifungal makes this unique liquid the perfect vaginal cleanse. It can be very difficult to identify the source of vaginal problems/diseases due to the fact that they could be bacterial, viral or fungal. Silver Sol vaginal cleansing destroys all these sources of vaginal disease. For these and many more reasons Silver Sol can cleanse multiple sources of vaginal disease including antibiotic resistant bacteria, STDs, yeast and do so safely as a liquid or gel.

The need for improved vaginal hygiene is evident when you research the sexually transmitted diseases, yeast infections, and occurrence of viral infections that cause cancer of the uterus and cervix. Silver Sol liquid destroys the cause of numerous vaginal diseases and will become a woman's best friend when it comes to itching, cramping and yeast infections.

SECTION V

The ESSENCE of Good Health

Silver Sol should be used as one part of a broader commitment to good health. Silver's benefits and effects are enhanced dramatically by what I call the ESSENCE of health. Each letter in the word determines one healthy principle.

E - eat correctly

S - sleep enough

S - supplement

E - exercise more

N - neutralize toxins

C - cleanse regularly

E - eliminate stress

If you perform one of these essential values you will receive a certain level of protection from disease and degeneration. However, by combining multiple values, your ability to prevent disease and promote wellness increases exponentially.

Exponential Benefit

In my dissertation research I examined exercise, nutrition, and the combination of both in preventing fatal viral infections. I discovered different types of exercise mobilize and activate the immune system, resulting in a 16 percent increase in immune cells. I also measured an 18 percent increase in the activity of immune cells (NK cells) due to herbal supplementation.

These benefits help a person function optimally and feel better. However, when a person exercised and took nutritional supplementation at the same time, they received an exponential increase in the number and activity of immune cells. When the protective levels of exercise were combined with the protective levels of nutritional supplementation, there was a 255 percent increase in the NK cells. These are the immune cells responsible for killing all foreign pathogens including fatal viruses and cancers.

I then combined exercise and nutritional supplementation together with a fatal virus (Cytomegalovirus CMV) to see if mice were able to prevent or survive a fatal viral challenge. Again, the principles of wellness were proven beneficial as the infected mice, who exercised on a treadmill and were fed nutritional supplements, survived a fatal viral infection. This experiment resulted in a 56 percent increase in the ability to survive a fatal viral infection, just by walking and taking nutritional supplements.

This example demonstrates how every healthy tool you give your body is one more level of protection. Adding multiple layers of protection increases your ability to prevent disease and promotes wellness.

Commitment to Good Health

A few years ago a chairperson for the National Institutes of Health's Anti-Viral Committee, Dr. Sidwell, caught a sinus infection that lingered for weeks and kept getting worse. He felt horrible—headaches, pain, fatigue, and sinuses that just wouldn't drain.

He went to his doctor and started antibiotics, and when they didn't work he started a stronger combination of antibiotics. That didn't work either, so he started using the anti-viral drugs he had developed. After some lab work it was determined that his sinus infection was resistant to all drugs. His doctor suggested surgery to keep the infection from going into his ears, eyes, and brain.

This was enough to scare him. At the time I was not aware of Silver Sol and its many benefits so I had suggested herbal supplements, exercise, and a good sleep system. He was not inclined to act until he heard the word "surgery." He took the herbs, rode a bike, and got some rest. Within three days his sinuses were completely clear—without the aid of drugs!

He was amazed. After all, he was the inventor of anti-viral drugs, and yet he avoided surgery with just supplements and exercise. All his years of wisdom convinced him that prevention was still the best answer. He continues to take supplements, exercise, and has water and air filters in his home.

From this experience I learned that, in addition to the above measures, family support has a profound impact on health. Dr. Sidwell is my father-in-law. It is scary to think that without his wife and children encouraging him to stick to a health regimen, the results may have been different. Fortunately, his family was firmly committed to the essence of good health.

Let's take a closer look at what it means to follow the ESSENCE of good health.

EAT CORRECTLY

The U.S. Department of Agriculture reports that 92 percent of Americans do not get sufficient nutrients from the foods they eat. Their dietary guidelines include balancing diet with exercise, eating grains with fruits and vegetables, eating a low fat diet, choosing a diet low in sugars, salt and alcohol, and not smoking or using tobacco.

To meet these guidelines, supplementation is needed—especially for children and the elderly. A child who doesn't receive proper nutrition will not achieve maximum physical and mental potential. The immune systems will not function correctly, bones don't grow properly and muscles are weak.

Most children develop their eating habits in the home and have established their eating and exercise habits by age 15. A recent report claims Americans are drinking more soda and eating less fresh whole foods. Those habits can carry on into later years. Here are the results from a recent survey of college students:

- 15 percent of college students did not eat any vegetables
- 40 percent ate a diet high in foods like French fries and ketchup, which they consider to be healthy forms of potatoes and tomatoes
- 20 percent did not consume any fruit

During the four years of college, the average girl gains 20 pounds. This diet shows one reason why. It has been reported that in the year 1900 the average person consumed 6-8 pounds of sugar per year. Today the estimate is over 200 pounds of sugar—and 1 in 13 adults is becoming diabetic in the process!

Conversely, there are tremendous benefits for those who consume natural fruit nectars and green drinks, eat vegetables, and keep sugar to a minimum. Adding fresh food to your diet provides antioxidants that neutralize toxins.

It is important to eat organic produce. Our fruits and vegetables are radiated with up to 30 million x-rays to stop the enzymes from softening fresh fruit. Genetically-altered fruits and vegetables can be detrimental to our health.

SLEEP ENOUGH

Sleep deprivation costs America an estimated 100 billion dollars a year in lost productivity, medical expenses, and sick leave time.

A National Sleep Foundation poll found the following:

- Nearly 7 out of 10 Americans said they experience sleep problems
- 69 percent of children have a sleep problem at least once a week
- 67 percent of elderly adults (40 and older) report frequent sleep problems

- 63 percent of adults do not get 8 hours of sleep a night (adults need 7-9 hours of sleep per night)
- 15 percent of adults have severe insomnia

When we don't get adequate sleep, we accumulate a sleep debt that can be difficult to pay back. If our sleep debt gets too high, we start to experience physical, emotional, and hormonal damage including high blood pressure, obesity, and mood and behavior changes.

In a study, 20-year-olds were only allowed to sleep four hours a night for seven days. At the end of the week they all tested positive for diabetes or hypoglycemia. This shows that lack of sleep can cause hormones to change.

How can you increase and improve your sleep? Exercise during the day helps exhaust your excess physical stress. A good diet can help you get better quality sleep which helps you feel better rested in the morning. Even a simple back massage can help relax the muscles and make going to sleep easier.

A schoolteacher and mother of four children didn't get more than five hours of sleep a night. Her family insisted something was wrong because she continued to gain weight, even when she ate half-meals. While visiting the doctor, she found she was insulin resistant and diabetic.

Her chiropractor recommended she take supplements, and walk 20 minutes every day. She was miraculously able to control her insulin levels without continued insulin injection, and within a year she lost 35 pounds.

SUPPLEMENT

As mentioned earlier, 92 percent of Americans do not get what they need from the foods they eat. There are more than 20,000 medical journal articles demonstrating the benefits of nutritional supplements. Even U.S. Public Law 103-417 states that the use of dietary supplements will prevent disease, promote wellness, and reduce long-term health care costs.

Silver Sol can be combined with any nutritional supplement, from herbs and antibiotics to pharmaceutical drugs. It should not, however, be combined with salt, as the chloride ion inactivates some of silver's effectiveness. After eating salty foods, wait one hour before using Silver Sol.

As detailed in the following section (EXERCISE MORE), supplementation can exponentially increase the effects of exercise and healthy living. Supplements can also benefit specific body systems such as gastrointestinal, immune, respiratory, and circulatory.

EXERCISE MORE

According to *Health and Hygiene Journal,* exercise helps prevent coronary heart disease, stroke, and some forms of cancer. Unfortunately, 6 out of 10 men and 7 out of 10 women are not sufficiently active to benefit their health, according to the Department of Health and CDC.

The average American has been gaining three pounds per year since the 1980s. More than 65 percent of us are overweight and 31 percent are obese, often due to lack of exercise and poor diet. The U.S. Health and Human Services Committee reports that obesity is the second leading cause of preventable death, with more than 300,000 obesity-related deaths each year.

The best solution for all of these problems is to walk 90 minutes a week. I recommend walking with weighted shoes, as it helps your legs grow stronger and helps you get exercise no matter what you're doing. If you walk five days a week you can realistically expect to burn 25 pounds of fat during the year.

I conducted research on the benefits of exercise in combination with nutritional supplements. Here's what I found:

By walking daily, you can increase the number of immune NK cells by about 15 percent. If you sprint for 10 seconds you can increase immune cells by about 23 percent. If you alternately walk and jog, you get about an 18 percent increase. This benefit lasts about four hours and offers added protection against viruses and abnormal cell growth.

I also tested what would happen if you only used a nutritional supplement and found that the activity of the immune cell increased by 18 percent. I found it remarkable that a supplement would activate the immune system.

I then combined exercise with nutritional supplementation and discovered a 255 percent increase in the number of NK cells. They continued to be active for 20 hours.

When you combine exercise with supplements you get an exponential benefit to the immune system that lasts five times longer. You should note that these are the immune cells that fight viruses and cancers best.

I wanted to see if this would prevent a fatal viral infection like the flu. When I infected mice with a fatal virus and then gave them supplements and exercised them on a treadmill, they developed a 64 percent increase in the ability to survive a fatal viral infection.

Here's the most important thing I learned from this process—exercise results in a mild benefit and supplement use results in a mild benefit. But when you combine the two, you increase the ability to fight off disease exponentially.

In addition to its benefit to the immune system, a new study also reports the benefits of exercise on depression. Those who exercised 90 minutes a week over a two-and-a-half month period were better able to control their depression more than by using tricyclic antidepressants (such as Prozac).

NEUTRALIZE TOXINS IN THE AIR AND WATER

The adult body is about 60 percent water and that of a child is 75 percent water. By the time we feel thirsty we are already dehydrated. Dehydration can cause dizziness, headache, dry mouth and tongue, confusion and incoherence. It is also the leading cause of hospitalization in those over 65.

To stay adequately hydrated, you must drink about 10 glasses of water per day. By drinking clean, pure water you can also help avoid excess body fat, poor muscle tone, constipation, toxic overload, and joint and muscle soreness.

Proper fluid intake is also a major key to weight loss. If you are dehydrated you will not lose fat. In fact, it takes 22 ounces of water to metabolize one ounce of fat. No water means no fat burning as your body is forced to use muscle for energy and to store fat.

Most of us don't realize that 90 percent of the time we think we are hungry, we are really just thirsty. The next time you are hungry in between meals, drink eight ounces of clean, pure water and wait 15 minutes. This will often curb your hunger.

Water Toxins

In America, 178 million people get their water from surface water systems and 85.9 million get it from ground water systems. This means that two thirds of Americans are really drinking water that was collected from the surface, i.e., the gutter. Forty percent of America is drinking water that is potentially unfit to drink!

Water helps convert food into energy. It also regulates body temperature, moistens the mouth, eyes, and nose and removes toxins through proper excretion. Contaminated water fills our bodies with toxins and can cause major diseases.

We should always try to drink optimized water. "Optimized" means that one oxygen molecule is combined with two hydrogen molecules and can transfer energy readily. The problem is that in tap water, for every one oxygen molecule, there are usually 36 hydrogen molecules clinging on and becoming free radicals once ingested.

Nine reasons to drink clean, pure, optimized water:

1. 75 percent of Americans are regularly dehydrated
2. 37 percent believe they are hungry when they are really thirsty because of toxins
3. A 3 percent dehydration results in slow metabolism (which means weight gain)
4. A 2 percent loss of body water results in short-term memory loss and trouble focusing
5. Children who don't absorb enough water are linked to obesity and reduced height
6. Water reduces cramps, fevers, and the craving for sweets
7. Water must be replenished every two hours
8. Dehydration is the number one reason for hospitalization among those 65 and older
9. Your body will take water out of your colon if you are dehydrated

Air Toxins

We spend 90 percent of our time inside. The EPA reports that 6 out of 10 buildings are contaminated with air pollution. These buildings can be 100 times more toxic than outdoor air. Toxins from carpet chemicals, cleansers, paint, glue, dust, and mold accumulate in your lungs, stick in your alveoli, and never come out again.

Some big cities have traffic and smog so thick it burns the eyes and clogs the lungs and skin pores. If you can smell the pollution in your hair as you wash it, just imagine the impact it is having on your lungs.

The Centers for Disease Control (CDC) recommends HEPA filters to remove bacteria and viruses. These filters are used in hospitals to keep doctors healthy despite being exposed to so many unhealthy people. These filters are especially beneficial in the winter months when bacteria spread is rampant.

CLEANSE

A clean home is a healthy home. This is the case for the human body as well. It requires regular cleansing of the intestines, blood, liver, and other vital organs. When the body is not clean, diseases begin to damage healthy tissues until eventually the systems of the body fail.

If you build a new wall over a wet and dirty area, mold can grow and eat away the newly formed walls. This is true with the intestinal system as well. If a person has a clogged intestine (constipation), no good thing can be absorbed. This leads to intestinal molds, yeasts, and other pathogens that damage the intestines and detoxification organs. When the intestines can't detoxify the fermenting foods fast enough, the extra burden falls on the liver and kidneys. These vital organs can perform very well, but only for a limited time. If the constipation continues, diseases can develop from chronic exposure to intestinal toxins.

With an intestinal cleanse, the body will be able to eliminate toxins from all systems of the body, including the brain. Without a regular cleanse, detoxification organs are overworked. Fermented sugars are stored in the muscles and the blood stream begins to circulate potentially pathogenic elements to all parts of the body.

No system of your body will work optimally if it is not cleansed regularly. You will heal faster, more completely, and with less inflammation if you consistently cleanse your intestines, blood, and liver.

ELIMINATE STRESS

The word stress comes from the Latin *strigi*, which means "to be drawn tight." Anyone who has experienced stress knows this is a very apt description.

There are four types of stress: eustress (good), distress (bad), hyperstress (too much), and hypostress (not enough). Regardless of the type, stress produces physical, psychological, emotional, and behavioral symptoms including:

- Racing heart
- Breathlessness
- Tight chest
- Dry mouth
- Indigestion
- Muscle twitches
- Frequent attacks of flu and sore throat
- Indecisiveness
- Poor concentration
- Bad dreams
- Sexual dysfunction
- Negative thoughts (including thoughts of suicide)
- Irritability
- Sleep disturbances
- Anger
- Blood sugar imbalances
- Low self-esteem
- Neglected self-care
- Tendency to avoid social activities
- Substance abuse
- Depression
- Lack of confidence

Stress is worse than you may think. In fact, some doctors believe stress is the major cause of all disease. It tears away at every body system, including your brain. Even worse, the stress of your past experiences also magnifies your reactivity to stress in the future.

Stress has a central command post—the hypothalamus, which regulates heart rate, blood pressure, and all involuntary bodily functions. Under long or extreme stress, the brain and its chemistry change, resulting in long- and short-term changes to behavior, personality, and even memory. Stress lowers natural immunity and allows damage to tissues, resulting in diseases such as rheumatoid arthritis and fibromyalgia. Stress also makes it hard to lose weight.

Fortunately, stress can be reduced and prevented and the symptoms can be reversed over time. A drink comprised of whole fruits can be used to protect the cellular DNA that might be damaged by cortisol. A supplement of omega-three fatty acids can protect the hypothalamus in the brain from becoming overworked, confused, or shutting down. A green drink can reduce the toxins from stress by helping them leave through the colon quickly. Each of these products contains antioxidants and can help reduce free radicals. When I travel to foreign countries, I experience jet lag and stress. I always try to sleep 12 hours and have a green drink to get me jump-started again.

WINNING THE WAR

The fight against disease is not a lost cause. I feel strongly that by combining healthy habits of ESSENCE with regular use of Silver Sol, the vast majority of contagious disease can be prevented and we can win the war. Let's now take a look at the wide range of Silver uses.

Endnotes

1. Clear Springs Press, Colloidal Silver

2. Fox, C.J. Jr., 1968. Silver sulfadiazine, a new topical therapy for Pseudomonas burns. Arch. Surg. 96:184-188.

3. Fox, C. J., 1969. Control of Pseudomonas infection in burns by Silver Sulfadiazine. Surg.Gynecol. Obstet. 128:1021-1026.

4. U.S House International Relations Committee, 2005. Written testimony on Black Mold and MRSA.

5. Illinois Institute of Technology. 2001. Anthrax.

6. Robinson, R., 2003. Bactericidal activity of ASAP Silver Solution on Yersinia Pestis, the etiological agent of plague. Department of Microbiology, Brigham Young University.

7. U.S. House Relations Committee. 2005. Written testimony on Malaria.

8. Hafkine, A., 2003. ASAP antiviral activity in Hepatitis B; DNA Polymerase Inhibition, Reverse Transcriptase Inhibition. Hafkine Institute for Training, Research and Testing.

9. Colloidal Silver: Medicinal Uses.

10. Carr, H., Wlodowski, T., 1973. Department of Microbiology, College of Physicians and Surgeons, Columbia University, New York, New York. Antimicrobial Agents and Chemotherapy. 10:585-587).

11. United States Patent Office. Patent # 7135195, Nov. 2006.

12. Merck Index., 1999. Silver. 1:645.

13. IRIS Report, 2005.

14. Healing capacity of Silver Sol in Pigs. University of Utah, 2005

15. Ghana Food and Drug Board New drug approval, 2007

16. EPA report and guidelines #D011

17. DeSouza, A. Current Science, 91(7), 2006. Bactericidal activity of combination of Silver-Water Dispersion with 19 antibiotics against seven microbial strains.

18. Institute for Antiviral Research. Silver Sol and H5N1 Influenza, 2005.

19. Nelson Labs, Brigham Young University. 2005.

20. Surgeons scrub test. 2005.

21. University of Cal Davis. Silver Sol and healthy intestinal flora. 2005.

22. Dr John R. Salzman, Radiation Oncologist)

23. General P.K.Carlton MD. Letter to the department of homeland security, 2007.

24. Orrin Hatch. Letter to Hon Tom Ridge Homeland Security, 2006.

25. Duan, L, et al. "Rapid and simultaneous detection of human hepatitis B virus and hepatitis C virus antibodies based on a protein chip assay using nano-gold immunological amplification and silver staining method." BMC Infect Dis. 2005 Jul 6;5:53.

26. Chang, AL, et al. "A case of argyria after colloidal silver ingestion." J Cutan Pathol. 2006 Dec;33(12):809-11.

27. Zeller, J.L. et al. "JAMA patient page. MSRA infections." JAMA. 2007 Oct 17; 298(15): 1826.

SECTION VI

GENERAL USES FOR BODY SYSTEMS

Silver Sol

Silver Sol may be your most effective tool to maintain, sustain and support your immune defenses.

General Usage:
- Maintenance dose: 1 teaspoon, hold under tongue for 30 seconds then swallow once a day
- Immune Support: 1 teaspoon, hold under tongue for 30 seconds then swallow, 3 times a day
- Acute Immune Issue: 2 teaspoons 2-3 times a day
- Chronic Immune Support: 1 teaspoon three times a day

Respiratory System:
- Respiratory Health: Swallow two teaspoons twice daily and spray 3-4 sprays in nose as needed.
- Nasal Health/Allergies: Swallow 2 teaspoons twice daily and spray into the nose 3-4 sprays 4 times a day.
- Mouth and Gum health: Hold 2 tablespoons in mouth and gargle for 4-5 minutes, then swallow. Twice daily.
- Throat Health: Hold 2 tablespoons in mouth for 3 minutes, then swallow; repeat several times a day. If using spray, 15 sprays every other hour.
- Lung Health: Swallow 2 tablespoons 2-3 times a day, and inhale 4 sprays four times a day.

Cardiovascular Health:
- 2 tablespoons, hold in mouth for 1 minute, then swallow, twice a day.

Digestive / Intestinal System:
- Gastrointestinal Health: Swallow two teaspoons twice daily.
- Intestinal Health Balance: Take 2 tablespoons of Silver Sol 2-3 times a day and combine with probiotics twice a day.

Urinary System:
- Drink 2 tablespoons twice daily.

Female Health:
- Use two to three ounces in affected area, hold for ten minutes then release, 1-2 times daily. And drink 2 tablespoons twice daily.

Sensory System:
- Ear Health: Point ear towards the sky and put 5 drops into ear and hold upright for 10 minutes. Repeat every 12 hours. And swallow 2 teaspoons twice daily.
- Eye Health: Use 1-2 drops every hour.

Immune/Allergy Health:
- Nasal Health/Allergies: Swallow 2 teaspoons twice daily and spray into the nose 3-4 sprays 1-4 times a day.

First Aid Recovery Support for Cuts, Scrapes, Bug Bites etc.:
- To support the immune system, swallow 2 teaspoons twice a day and apply gel topically as needed.

Skin and Nails:
- Skin Health: To support the immune system, apply gel twice daily or as needed, and swallow liquid 2 teaspoons twice daily.
- Nail Fungus: Frequent use of small amounts of product is best.

Healthy Water:
- 2 tablespoons per gallon of water. Wait 4 minutes and drink as needed.

Traveling:
- 1 teaspoon before, during and after flying or driving, for general immune support. Hold under tongue for 30 seconds before swallowing. And spray 3-4 sprays into nose before flying.

Please be aware that federal regulations limit dietary supplements to oral administration even if structure function claims may be specific to certain body parts.

Note: *These statements have not been evaluated by the FDA. This product is not intended to cure, treat, diagnose or prevent any disease.*

Immune System

Silver Sol is a mild immune modulator. It has been shown to cause an increase in the number and activity of immune cells when taken orally. This means that if you drink a teaspoon of Silver Sol liquid twice daily you will find an increase in the number of white blood cells, which destroy foreign pathogens in the body. It should be noted that this improvement in immune health occurs within an hour after drinking Silver Sol and will last for approximately 24-48 hours after. You should expect to have improved defenses against bacteria viruses and yeast during the time you are taking Silver Sol and for a day or two after. In addition Silver Sol can help protect and shield the body from diseases caused by these pathogens by killing them upon direct contact.

Recommendations:

Drink one teaspoon 2 times daily to support immune function, and apply Silver Sol gel as needed to affected areas that require gel application. Benefits can be measured in the blood within one hour and will last up to two days after the last drink. Benefits from the gel can be felt in 3-5 minutes as it helps reduce pain and inflammation. For more serious health concerns Silver Sol liquid can be taken 2-4 times greater doses.

Respiratory System

Silver Sol destroys bacteria viruses and yeast that resides in or around the respiratory system (ears, nose, throat, lungs).

Recommendations:

- Inhaled (from a nebulizer 30 minutes a day or two episodes of 15 minutes each).
- Drink two teaspoons twice a day, or spray fine mist up nose 2-5 times a day.
- Apply gel to the nose, sinuses mouth, and hands to prevent infections or spread of germs. This can be done 1-5 times a day or as often as it takes to keep the nasal passages moist.

Reproductive System

Silver Sol benefits the reproductive organs by destroying bacteria, viruses and yeast that may cause damage to the delicate organs and tissues of the reproductive system. Silver destroys bacteria that cause urinary tract infections and yeast that causes yeast infections. This is accomplished in about ten minutes as long as the silver comes in close proximity to the germs.

Recommendations:

- Drink Silver Sol liquid two teaspoons twice a day to help destroy germs from the inside out.
- Apply Silver Sol gel to the reproductive tissues that are susceptible to infections (vagina, penis, foreskin, breast, pubic hair etc,). This should be done twice a day or more often if needed.
- Apply the Silver Sol gel to a tampon and insert for 90 minutes in order to stay in contact with germs intra-vaginally.
- Apply the gel twice a day to the foreskin, condom or genitals to protect yourself or your sex partner.

Circulatory System

Silver Sol destroys the bacteria the causes cardiovascular diseases. The gel can be used as a toothpaste to kill the bacteria that causes bad breath, cavities, abscesses, and heart disease because this kind of bacteria resides in the gums. A mouthwash twice a day will kill bacteria in the mouth as well.

Digestive System

Silver Sol liquid and gel can be swallowed and enter the digestive tract where it will destroy bacteria, viruses an yeast. There are serious diseases that originate in the intestines, colon, and vital organs of digestion. Silver Sol can pass through the digestive tract unchanged. This means the silver kills germs in the kidneys and bladder just as effectively as it kills bacteria in the mouth. This is significant because kidney, liver and bladder infections are very difficult to control but silver will pass through the blood stream and flow through the liver thus cleansing the germs out of the liver, then pass through the kidneys and on to the bladder where pathogens will be destroyed when they come in close proximity with the silver nano-particles.

Recommendations:
- Drink two teaspoons of Silver Sol twice daily for digestive health. In the event there is a food poisoning, diarrhea, or other digestive malady, silver liquid can be swallowed one ounce every hour for 12 hours or until remedied. Usually the most serious symptoms of the food poisoning problem can be brought under control in 2-4 hours with the remainder of the sickness requiring maintenance doses (two teaspoons twice daily).
- Apply the gel to any orifice of the body that may need protection from germs (1-4 times a day).

Hair Skin and Nails

Silver Sol liquid and gel destroy the bacteria, viruses and yeast that cause diseases in the hair, skin and nails. The liquid can be used in shampoo, lotions, gels, and moisturizers and under nails. The gel can be applied to all skin conditions and can be pushed under nails to destroy yeast.

Recommendations:
- All of these can benefit from drinking Silver Sol liquid two teaspoons twice a day and applying the gel 2-4 times a day or as needed topically.

SECTION VII

SILVER USES A-Z

Abscesses

Because it's an open wound, an abscess can expose the blood flow to possible bacterial contamination. It is very important to kill the bacteria in the wound.

Silver Sol can be used as a mouth rinse for an abscess in the mouth. Hold one ounce of liquid in your mouth for at least six minutes, two to three times a day. It can then be swallowed, providing an internal rinse as well.

You can also use liquid Silver Sol as a rinse for an abscess on the outside of your body. When you first clean the abscess, rinse it with liquid Silver Sol. If it requires a bandage, soak the gauze bandage in liquid Silver Sol and put a drop of gel on the surface before taping it into place.

For a very small abscess, you can simply put a drop of the Silver Sol gel on a Band-Aid and place it over the abscess. For a large abscess, spray the gel or the liquid Silver Sol on the wound one to four times a day.

Aches

Aches can occur from inflammation within a joint, muscle, or body system, like the intestinal or cardiovascular system. Silver Sol has the ability to destroy the cause of inflammation—bacteria, viruses, parasites, and even yeast in some cases.

By killing the cause, inflammation can be reduced, maintained, and even prevented. Just take one teaspoon of Silver Sol one to three times a day. Using glucosamine, condroitant sulfate, and MSM also helps aches. In addition, silver has the ability to help modulate the cause of pain in a very mild manner.

Acid Reflux

Acid reflux is also referred to as heartburn. It occurs when too much stomach acid pools in the stomach and then returns back into the throat or mouth. The associated pain is a result of the hydrochloric acid dissolving and digesting the normal tissues of the esophagus, mouth, and throat.

To stop the problem, it is necessary to stop the flow of acid. One way is to take digestive enzymes and neutralize those acids. Another way is to take antacids which help absorb those acids and pass them through your digestive tract.

Silver Sol can be taken daily to help the burns caused by the acid. Take one to two teaspoons, two to five times a day as needed. In addition, you can take acidophilus or digestive enzymes, which help transport stomach acids out of the body. As a last resort, a physician can pre-scribe acid blockers or drugs that will stop the production of acid in the stomach.

A young woman in her early 20s was taken to the emer-gency room, thinking she might be having a heart attack. After being checked for all the signs and symptoms, a heart attack was ruled out. Yet she was still doubled over in pain and having stabbing pains right over her heart. She was given a cocktail of antacids and pain relievers, and within a few minutes the pain subsided. The doctors deduced that it was not a heart attack, but acid reflux.

Two weeks later she was in the same situation, experiencing the same stabbing pain. Because she knew it was acid re-

flux, she went to the store and bought over-the-counter acid blockers. This worked for about six months.

She had to keep increasing the quantity and frequency of her acid blocker use to find relief. She soon noticed a sore throat that she just couldn't get rid of. It became so bothersome that she went back to the doctor.

The doctor found that her sore throat was caused by acid reflux. The acid had been traveling from her stomach up to her throat, literally dissolving the back of her throat. Acid reflux is strong enough to dissolve your esophagus to the point that surgery is needed to repair the damage. Luckily she caught it in time.

This young woman also had a lot of fever blisters. When she would lie down at night, the acid would reflux up her esophagus and into her mouth. The acid would start to burn little holes in her mouth and cause cankers. If you frequently have cankers, it may be from acid reflux. To find relief, you should utilize silver, digestive enzymes, and acidophilus on a regular basis.

Acne

Acne attacks people of all ages, from infants to adults. Acne can be caused by bacteria getting inside of a hair follicle or a sweat gland called a sebaceous gland. Once the bacteria gets under the skin it will duplicate itself, dissolving healthy tissue in the process and leaving scars behind. To get rid of the acne, you must get rid of the bacteria.

To kill the bacteria, take two teaspoons of silver twice a day. Silver should also be applied topically twice a day.

You can expect to see reduction in the size and in the damage of the acne within 24 hours. Total improvement of the skin will take about four weeks—the amount of time necessary for new skin to grow from the bottom to the top layer.

Antibiotics and Silver

Dr. Rustum Roy published an article in *Current Science* medical journal about silver. His findings showed Silver Sol can improve healing functions because it is a broad-spectrum microbial, similar in results to any pharmaceutical grade antibiotic—without causing resistance, mutation, or tolerance like antibiotics.

An antibiotic can only be taken for about two weeks before bacteria mutate and become resistant to the drug. For this reason, antibiotics can't be used on a continuous basis for prevention. Silver Sol creates no resistance and can be taken every day. In addition, antibiotics only work on a narrow range of bacteria; silver has a very broad range of use.

When antibiotics are supplemented with Silver Sol the benefits can be as much as tenfold. Use silver daily for prevention. If a crisis occurs, antibiotics can be added. The silver will destroy the bacteria that the antibiotic misses.

Attention Deficit Disorder

Though we are unsure of all the causes and types of Attention Deficit Disorder (ADD), we do know that sugar can be a trigger and certain drugs, vaccinations, and lack of sleep may all play a role as well.

In the event of ADD, it is important to reduce sugar, cleanse the intestinal system, and restore proper function to the brain with B vitamins, lecithin, phosphatidyl serine, and essential fatty acids. Drinking two teaspoons of Silver Sol twice a day will kill bacteria, viruses, and mold, and reduce the neurotoxins sent to the brain.

Age Spots

Age spots develop when the liver doesn't produce enough enzymes to detoxify what is circulating through the blood stream. Certain toxins can be deposited in the fats underneath your skin, creating an age spot—usually a permanent effect like a tattoo.

You can get the liver working properly again, and get the proper production of enzymes at the same time, by drinking liquid Silver Sol on a regular basis. Putting Silver Sol gel on the age spot can help excrete that which has been stored under the skin. For the best benefit, apply topically two to four times a day and take one teaspoon orally twice a day.

Aging

There are many reasons why we may age prematurely—a liver that doesn't function properly, tissues that degenerate too quickly, a sedentary lifestyle, lack of nutrients, and the toxins that are all around us.

Yeast is one of the main components in premature aging. We have yeast between our toes and in our intestines. It's found anywhere there is a warm, moist area and destroys one cell at a time. Likewise, bacteria can cause tissue damage. Silver prevents premature aging by killing bacteria, viruses, and yeast.

Drink one teaspoon of liquid Silver Sol twice a day for wellness and prevention. If you are sick, drink two teaspoons twice a day. Silver Sol gel can also be applied to specific areas topically one to three times a day. Additional benefits can come from using freeform amino acids, vitamins, minerals, and essential fatty acids.

A research project was conducted to see if Silver Sol could help prevent aging in roses. Eighteen roses were clipped from the same bush. The leaves were stripped off and each rose was placed in its own vase. Each vase contained water; half of the vases also contained Silver Sol liquid.

The roses placed only in water died in a week-and-a-half. The roses supplemented with Silver Sol were in bloom and fully healthy for three-and-a-half weeks. Silver Sol helped prolong the life of a rose by at least 200%. And surprisingly, the roses in the Silver Sol liquid re-grew their leaves. Silver Sol not only helped prevent the aging process from taking place, it demonstrated regenerative properties with new leaves growing where the old leaves had been stripped off.

Allergies

Allergies occur when an allergen triggers an allergic response in the body. The immune system mobilizes and activates, causing inflammation, swelling, and mucus production. When this happens in the throat or the sinuses, it results in a sore throat or sinus infection. This can lead to coughing, sneezing, irritation in our lungs and even asthma-like symptoms.

The first step to improving asthma symptoms is to remove the allergen—e.g., the pollen, the dust, or irritating laundry detergent. While we can't remove all the allergens from our air or water, we can remove a lot of bacteria, viruses, and mold from inside our body by drinking liquid Silver Sol. We can protect the outside of our body by using Silver Sol gel topically.

To fight allergies, drink one teaspoon in the morning and one at night. Spraying silver into the nasal cavities will also reduce swelling and congestion. Nebulized silver can be inhaled a total of 30 minutes each day and gel can be applied inside the nostrils to counteract skin irritation.

Alzheimer's Disease

Alzheimer's disease causes the brain to slowly loose function. There are many suspected causes, from heavy metal toxicity to inflammation. According to the MERK Index medical journal, silver is the one metal that is not classified as a heavy metal. It will not accumulate in the brain like lead does. In fact, Silver Sol has been used in combination with freeform amino acids and phosphatidyl serine to help improve circulation and mental memory and function. Taking one teaspoon of Silver Sol morning and evening will destroy intestinal neurotoxins that cause inflammation of the brain.

Anti-Aging
(See Aging)

Anti-Bacterial

Found on the skin, in the blood stream, in the intestines, or in the hair, bacteria cause countless diseases. When serious diseases are examined in the lab they find that every serious chronic disease is associated with the presence of pleiomorphic bacteria or mold. These damage the immune function that normally protects the cell from foreign invaders. When the bacteria or mold invade a cell and reduce the immune protection, they allows toxins and contagions to enter the cell and damage the DNA, allowing serious disease to originate. Silver Sol starts killing bacteria in as little as fifteen seconds. If you put Silver Sol gel, liquid, or mist in direct contact with bacteria, the bacteria will usually be totally destroyed within six minutes. Some bacteria may take longer but can be destroyed with regular Silver Sol use.

For preventive use, drink one teaspoon of Silver Sol each morning and night. That dose can be doubled to fight an aggressive bacterial infection. It may be applied topically to any affected areas one to four times a day. Immune-supporting herbs may also be used.

> *Nursing home residents often have a weakened immune system. This makes them susceptible to bacterial infections. Many develop bedsores, and bacteria—like staph—will get into the sore. Bedsores can last up to seven years without healing. Imagine having an open wound, living in a nursing home, and having an infection that is treated with antibiotics that stop working after just a few weeks.*
>
> *Silver Sol gel is currently being used in clinical trials. Results are showing that it can help close deep open-tunneling wounds, leprosy, and staph, including MRSA. By spraying the gel on the wound twice a day, bacteria are destroyed and the body can heal itself more quickly.*

Anti-Fungal

Fungus can get into any warm, moist area and often feeds off of sugars. Cutting off sugars can combat intestinal fungus or yeast. For a yeast or fungus infection in the armpits or vagina, apply Silver Sol directly to the yeast or take liquid Silver Sol internally. It can be applied topically one to four times a day, or as needed. The recommend liquid use is two teaspoons, one to three times a day. Acidophilus supplementation may be used simultaneously.

Yeast and fungus can get inside your intestines, causing muscle pain and symptoms of depression and attention deficit disorder. It can also result in all the symptoms of headaches, lymph problems, lupus and autoimmune disorders, including fibromyalgia.

Many people have resolved these symptoms by taking two teaspoons of Silver Sol daily as part of an intestinal yeast and fungus cleanse. The cleanse may be accompanied by one to three weeks of flu-like symptoms while the yeast leaves the body. Silver Sol Colonics have been used in the rectum, and douches are being successful in the vagina.

Anti-Tumor

Tumors can have a myriad of causes. Tumors are almost always caused by a combination of problems. One bacterium is not usually the cause of a tumor, but when bacteria get into the cell and neutralize your immune function, you become more susceptible to other toxins in the air and water. This allows DNA to be damaged and a tumor to form. Bacteria such as hepatitis B can cause cancer. Viruses can also cause tumors and cancer, including the human papilloma virus that can result in cervical cancer in women.

Those with a tumor should drink one to four ounces of Silver Sol liquid a day, sipping the Silver Sol every hour for the first 4-8 hours. Drink two ounces a day for the next five days—two tablespoons in the morning and two tablespoons in the night. Apply topically two to three times a day to the tumor if it is visible. In addition, you may find an intestinal cleansing daily with milk thistle beneficial. For more acute problems, drink four ounces one day and sip it every hour the next day.

If cancer runs in the immediate family, two tablespoons of Silver Sol in the morning and evening can be used as a preventive method.

Maintaining a diet that is low in fat and sugar, and high in proteins, fiber, fruits and vegetables will also help. In addition you want to get at least eight hours of sleep a night. You'll also want to take supplements that have immune enhancing capabilities. You want to exercise if possible on a daily basis. I'm not talking strenuous, but just a walking type of exercise to make sure your circulation is good and your body's immune function is properly working in concert with your lymph system. You want to neutralize toxins in your air and water using proper filtration in your home. You want to cleanse the intestines and your blood. You cleanse the intestines with an intestinal cleanse, you cleanse your liver by using milk thistle on a daily basis in a supplement form, then you cleanse the blood stream by taking a large amount of antioxidants. And you want to eliminate as much stress as you possibly can.

Anti-Viral

Viruses cause many diseases that we don't have pharmaceutical drugs to cure. For this reason, the human race is at a high risk for virus activity. We have viruses that are being treated incorrectly with antibiotics. Antibiotics do nothing to destroy or cure viral infections. Silver Sol is very powerful and patented against both reverse transcriptase and DNA polymerase viruses, interfering with their replication process.

By drinking two tablespoons of Silver Sol in the morning and night, you can potentially defeat an existing viral infection. Inhaling a nebulized form of silver works best for a viral infection in the lungs or sinuses. Drops can also be placed in your ears, eyes, nose, or throat twice a day.

To prevent a cold or flu, drink one teaspoon twice a day. If you are exposed to a lot of coughing and sneezing, the dose can be doubled. Immune-stimulating herbs are also beneficial.

Antibiotic Alternative

According to Dr. Rustum Roy (Penn State University) Silver Sol is more broad-spectrum than anything found in the drug world or nature. This means Silver Sol kills more than just a tiny segment of bacteria, like antibiotics do. Silver Sol kills all the bacteria except the healthy (probiotic) bacteria. This can happen because the healthy flora (lactobacillus) secretes a protective layer or lactobacillus around itself to protect against the acidic stomach acids. This protective layer prohibits the silver from rupturing the cell membrane because it cannot penetrate through the lactobacillus outer coating. This is demonstrated when a person takes antibiotics, and the action of the drugs kill the healthy flora, resulting in diarrhea. This is not seen when a person takes a quadruple dose of Silver Sol. In fact I have swallowed 8 ounces at one time (a 48 times normal dose) and never produced diarrhea. Remember it is the Silver Sol that improves antibiotic function and makes antibiotics up to ten fold stronger when taken with Silver Sol. It should be noted that a person taking Silver Sol daily (1 teaspoon 1-3 times a day) should destroy bacterium, viruses and yeast that cause the majority of illnesses, so you may never need to take an antibiotic again. According to a study performed by Nelson Labs, Silver Sol was found to completely kill all tested bacteria and cause NO resistance. This is important because it proves that Silver Sol is not going to cause the bacteria to get stronger or have the problems that plague antibiotic drugs.

Appetite Suppressant

Many people who suffer from overeating say they just can't seem to satisfy their appetite. Food craving can be increased by an intestinal yeast growth that puts neurotoxins into the blood stream. This creates damage everywhere the blood circulates, including the brain. Yeast is fed by sugar, and causes the body to crave more sugar.

Silver Sol will not directly control your appetite nor suppress it. However, if you have a yeast infection, Silver Sol can kill the yeast in your intestines, decreasing neurotoxins and food craving.

Silver Sol should be considered for any dietary plan. One teaspoon twice a day will help maintain wellness. A digestive cleanse will also be beneficial.

Arthritis

Arthritis is characterized by painful swelling and inflammation in the joints. This can happen when uric acid is not excreted from the body quickly enough and is deposited in the joints of the toe, ankle, or knee. It can recrystalize, creating the same effect has having sand crystals between your joints. This damages the joint directly, causing inflammation around the joint and inflaming muscles, tendons, and cartilage.

By drinking two teaspoons twice a day, or as needed, Silver Sol can help reduce pain and inflammation. Silver Sol gel can be applied topically to the joint if it is hot or red. Glucosamine, chondroitin sulfate, and essential fatty acids may also be used.

Asthma

Asthma occurs when the bronchioles—the breathing tubes of the body and lungs—become inflamed and swell shut, preventing the body from drawing oxygen into the lungs. This results in choking, coughing, and heavy mucus production that can clog the breathing tubes to the point of asphyxiation.

To reduce inflammation, inhale Silver Sol from a nebulizer for 15 minutes in the morning and at a night. One teaspoon of Silver Sol liquid should also be taken twice a day. The gel can be placed inside the nostrils as a lubricant to help prevent against triggers for an asthma attack. Probiotics can also help reduce inflammation that originates from the digestive tract.

Athlete's Foot

Athlete's foot is basically a fungal infection on the skin. It occurs when we put our feet in shoes and keep them in a warm, moist area where fungus can grow. The first step to prevention is to wear clean shoes and reduce the amount of time that your foot stays in a moist sock.

Silver Sol can be sprayed into your socks or directly on the foot. Silver Sol gel is an even better option in this situation. It can be applied between the toes to kill any yeast growth. You can also spray silver into your shoes to kill any bacteria. In addition to athlete's foot, fungus can get underneath your toenails. By soaking your feet for 30 minutes every other day in a Silver Sol bath, you will kill the toenail fungus and the athlete's foot. The fungus will return if you continue to wear shoes or socks that are housing bacteria or fungus.

By killing the bacteria and yeast, Silver Sol will also remove the odor associated with athlete's foot.

Autism

We don't know all the causes of autism. It affects people of all ages, but seems to develop early in life. Autism has also been associated with some vaccinations and inoculations. Antioxidants will help improve an autistic situation.

One class of autistic children who drank one teaspoon of Silver Sol morning and night showed improved behavior, were less irritated and agitated, learned better, and asked more intellectual questions. Though it did not cure their autism, it did improve their symptoms. Children weighing more than 75 pounds should take two teaspoons morning and night. Probiotics, arginine supplementation, and phosphatitle serine may also help.

Backache

Silver Sol has been shown to improve backaches associated with or caused by irritations on the skin or muscle tension. Applying the gel one to four times a day can help reduce pain and inflammation. Silver Sol will not help a backache caused by bone problems.

Bacteria

Bacteria are single cell organisms that actually grow within or outside your body. Left uninhibited, bacteria can cause disease or death. Many of today's health problems result from bacteria. Pneumonia, one of the leading causes of death in America, comes from bacteria inside of the lungs.

Silver Sol will destroy bacteria in approximately six minutes. You will feel the effects within the first two hours of use and the benefits will continue as long as you use the product. Silver Sol should also be combined with vitamins, minerals, essential fatty acids, amino acids, and antioxidants.

Bacterial Infections
(See Anti-Bacterial)

Bad Breath

Bad breath is usually caused by bacteria residing in the mouth and gums or between the teeth. Using Silver Sol rinse can destroy these bacteria. By rinsing the mouth for six minutes in the morning and at night, you will get rid of the bad breath.

Bad breath can also be caused by strep throat or a staph infection. In these cases, bacteria destroy the healthy tissue, causing red blisters and white pus to form in the back of throat. The odor comes as a result of the degenerating tissue. Silver Sol is the fastest way to remedy the problem.

Spraying Silver Sol into the nose four times a day can treat odor caused by a sinus infection.

Bedsores

When a bed does not have proper balance, pressure points can form. Irritation or rashes on the skin then lead to open wounds. To treat bedsores, get a good bed with a neutral balance. Do not use too much laundry detergent on bedding and sheets.

Silver Sol gel can be applied directly to the bedsore one to four times a day. The gel should be kept in place with a sterile bandage. You can expect improvement to begin very quickly after Silver Sol is introduced to a wound. Improvement in diabetics may take two to three times longer because of circulation problems.

Black Mold

Black mold is a fungus or yeast that grows in wet areas of the home like showers or walls. The mold will release spores into the air. If these spores reach your lungs, they will produce asthma- and chronic fatigue-like symptoms.

To remove the mold, spray liquid Silver Sol on it and let it stand for 10 minutes before wiping it off. This will destroy the mold and likely prevent it from re-growing.

Bladder Infection

Urine remains in the bladder for about six hours before it is drained. If bacteria get into the bladder, they will duplicate every 20 minutes—a bladder infection can become serious very quickly. The infection will degrade the lining of the bladder and possibly travel up the tubes from the bladder to the kidneys, causing a kidney infection.

To treat a bladder infection, two tablespoons of Silver Sol should be taken hourly for the first two days. For the next two weeks, take two tablespoons twice a day. You should expect to destroy the bladder infection within the first 12 to 24 hours.

Silver Sol liquid can be taken with cranberry juice or juniper berries.

I was on a trip to Asia when I got a bladder infection. I didn't have access to Silver Sol for about 24 hours. In that time, my bladder infection progressed from burning when I urinated, to passing blood.

I went to the doctor to find out what type of bacterial infection I had, so I could know what kind of antibiotics to take. Twelve hours before my doctor's appointment I started taking Silver Sol liquid. I drank one ounce each hour for four hours and then went to two teaspoons twice a day.

By the time I got to the doctor and gave a urine sample, I was bacteria free. There was a hint of blood, but no bacteria. The doctors were absolutely baffled by how such a severe bladder infection could be cleared up so quickly. The answer was simple. I took a large amount of Silver Sol liquid and it destroyed the bacteria in my bladder. The doctor said I didn't even need to take antibiotics.

If you have bleeding or serious pain during urination, it is important to see a doctor.

Body Odor

Since most body odor is caused by bacteria, Silver Sol can help control the production of odor. Spray or apply silver to the affected area and drink one teaspoon twice daily. This can also help with bad breath.

Blood Cleanser

Bacteria, viruses, yeast, parasites, and other toxins can get inside our blood. Silver Sol is one of the best tools for blood cleansing. It will enter a single red blood cell and cleanse at the cell level.

For acute blood cleansing, take one ounce every hour for four hours. For some serious conditions, you will need to take one four ounce bottle every day for the first three days, followed by a maintenance dose of two tablespoons twice a day.

To cleanse your blood each day, take one to two teaspoons, one to three times a day. Vitamin E in soft gel form may also help.

Boils

Boils occur when bacteria or viruses get under the skin and duplicate, destroying the healthy tissue. The duplication produces a pustule, which is similar to cystic acne, only it doesn't need a hair follicle or sebaceous gland to get down into the skin. Boils can be caused by simple irritations such as the rubbing of a belt on the skin or agitation on the side of a foot.

A boil can be treated by applying Silver Sol gel topically one to four times a day. In some cases, you may want to cover the boil with a bandage. In addition, you will want to drink two teaspoons of Silver Sol liquid twice a day.

As soon as the liquid and the gel come in contact with the bacteria, the boil growth will stop. Within about two hours you'll feel inflammation reduction. You will see improvement of the boil within four hours.

Bones

Bones can have a number of problems—breaks, infections, stoppage in the production of bone marrow and red blood cells—and pain is almost always associated with these problems. Silver Sol liquid taken on a daily basis can help reduce the bacteria, virus, and mold within the system, thus reducing the impact on the bones.

Silver Sol can help reduce the infection rate associated with broken bones or compound fractures, allowing the immune system to repair the bone much quicker. Calcium and magnesium may also be used.

Bowels

Bowels can have a lot of problems—from constipation and colitis to infections, diarrhea, and yeast infections. Taken regularly, Silver Sol liquid can help destroy the bacteria and yeast that cause many of these problems.

While regular cleanses are very efficient at removing constipation and toxins, often they do not remedy the cause of the problem, which may be yeast or bacteria. Silver Sol can help destroy the cause of the problem. You should expect to see benefits within the first two days.

Brain Cleansing

It is very difficult to get cleansing agents across the blood/brain barrier, but there are cases where the brain needs cleansing. The first step is to take white refined sugar out of your diet. The second step is to inhale Silver Sol liquid from a nebulizer. This allows the silver to travel through the nasal passages and lungs into the brain quicker and easier than through the blood stream. Inhale the mist 30 minutes a day and take two teaspoons of Silver Sol twice a day.

Breast Cancer

Breast cancer can be caused by high levels of bad estrogens, toxins, radiation, and many other problems. It has been estimated that as many as 60 percent of all cancers have a bacterial cause.

Drinking Silver Sol in the following doses can help prevent bacteria from causing cancer: Four ounces day one and four more ounces day two, sipping it every hour; two ounces a day for the next five days.

Drink two tablespoons in the morning and two tablespoons at night for maintenance. You can apply the Silver Sol gel topically two to three times a day as well. Antioxidants will also be beneficial.

Radiation treatment can burn the skin. Applying Silver Sol gel to the affected area will help prevent cellular damage and reduce pain.

Bronchitis

Bronchitis can be bacterial or a virus that causes the inflammation of the bronchioles—the tubes that the pass air from the throat down into the lungs. Bronchitis results in excess mucus production, clogged lungs, and coughing.

Bronchitis can be cleared up by drinking two teaspoons of Silver Sol two to four times a day, inhaling from a nebulizer 15 minutes twice a day, and by using an intra-nasal spray twice a day for congestion.

For those living, working, or traveling with someone with bronchitis, spray Silver Sol into the nose for prevention. The gel can also be applied to the inside of the nostrils. Immune-stimulating herbs and co-enzyme Q10 will also help. A cellular cleanse will prevent toxins and bacteria and viruses from gaining access blood stream.

Bruises

Bruises occur when a blood vessel is ruptured and blood pools in the tissue around it. Bruising often results from impact, but can also be caused by bacterial or viral infections. It can also occur when blood doesn't clot well.

Silver Sol helps remove the blood from the tissue, improving the bruise. Simply soak a sterile bandage in liquid silver and place it on the bruise. Silver Sol gel can also be applied to the wound one to four times a day.

A few years back, I injured myself very badly. I broke the orbital bone over my eye and had to have 15 stitches. This resulted in the biggest black eye I had ever seen. My eye was swollen shut. The bruise was dark purple because veins had ruptured around my eye.

I applied Silver Sol gel four times a day and took two teaspoons of Silver Sol liquid twice a day. The attending physician, Colonel Molof, a top military doctor, said it healed three times faster than any comparable wound he'd ever seen.

The injury healed so quickly because the gel killed all of the bacteria and mold that may have been impeding the immune system from doing its job. Silver Sol also reduces inflammation at the same time.

Bug Bites

When you get bitten by a bug or stung by a bee, toxins are introduced into your system. Silver Sol helps by reducing inflammation and pain and improves wound healing. A bandage soaked in Silver Sol can be applied directly to the bite. Drinking one ounce of Silver Sol liquid twice a day for two days will also lessen tissue damage and improve toxin excretion. You can expect faster improvement and less inflammation.

Burns

Burns occur from the sun, radiation, x-rays, fire, heat, and from other chemicals in our environment. Silver Sol is at its very best when it's used to treat a burn. It reduces pain and inflammation and improves wound healing. Silver Sol liquid can be sprayed on the burn or used to soak the burn, and the gel can be applied to the wound where a significant reduction in pain, inflammation and tissue damage will be visible in the first hour.

Often burn wounds are so painful that you will want to spray on Silver Sol liquid or gel. The gel will stay on the wound for a long period of time. The liquid will get into the wound very quickly, but needs to be reapplied every few hours. Drink one ounce of Silver Sol liquid twice a day until the burn is gone.

I know a fair-skinned young man who went to the beach and got very badly sunburned. We took a photo of his face and then applied the Silver Sol gel to just one half of his face. This would allow him to see the effects of Silver Sol as compared to his untreated skin.

The gel side did not ever blister, the redness faded quickly and the pain was resolved in minutes. The untreated side of his face blistered and peeled, taking about a week-and-a-half to heal. It was painful, red, and irritated. Silver Sol works on the worst of burns.

An 80-year-old woman suffered third degree burns when a pot of coffee fell in her lap. The wounds from her thigh to her knee were so deep she could not even receive a skin graft. Her doctors were considering surgery to deal with the burn.

Instead they took a chance and tried Silver Sol gel. The gel was sprayed on twice a day. In 66 days she was absolutely healed. The wounds had become absolutely scar-free, with just a few lines showing where she had been burned. Equally important, she did not have to take pain-killing drugs throughout the process.

Cancer

While silver has proven promising against many health conditions, those who have cancer or who may suspect they have cancer should always consult a physician before pursuing any course of treatment.

Cancer is always caused by a multiplicity of factors. Toxins, poisons, and pesticides have all been proven to cause cancers. Bacteria are one of the greatest causes of cancer because it neutralizes your immune system, allowing damage inside the cell on the DNA level. It is estimated that up to 60 percent of all cancers have a root in bacterial causes.

Silver Sol is a broad-spectrum preventive agent. It destroys bacteria in as little as 15 seconds and kills the viruses and mold that may also cause cancer.

Those suffering from cancer should drink four ounces of Silver Sol on day one and four ounces on day two, sipping it every hour. Drink two ounces a day for the next five days; take two tablespoons twice a day thereafter as a maintenance dose.

Sinus, mouth, throat, or lung cancer patients may want to use an inhaled form of liquid Silver Sol. One ounce can be inhaled from a nebulizer 30 minutes a day. This allows the Silver Sol to come in deep contact with the lungs, bronchioles, and sinuses. This approach should be combined with oral Silver Sol use.

There is also a very experimental method for IV usage. About 3,000 cases have used Silver Sol intravenously, with no reported toxicity problems. An IV can be made utilizing 250 CCs of Silver Sol liquid at 10 parts per million. Mix one to one with a D5W mixture hung in a bag and dripped for one hour, given every other day for 10 total doses.

It should be noted that saline solution cannot be used because the salts in the saline inactivate the Silver Sol. This is a very important formulation and can be adjusted in any parts per million of the Silver Sol. Using the mathematical proportion of 250 CCs, you can use any part per million that you need to begin with.

When you put Silver Sol liquid directly in the veins it will begin killing even the most serious bacteria in 15 seconds. Noticeable improvements will occur within the first two days. It has shown to be promising against viral infections like hepatitis, against cancer, and even against Epstein-Barr and the AIDS virus. Milk thistle can be used as a liver and intestinal cleanse. Drinking antioxidants daily will help cleanse the blood as well.

Silver and Cellular Abnormalities

According to the *Journal of Chem. Medicinal Chem.* (Nov. 2007), beams of ultraviolet light can be used to destroy tumors and cancers. Special molecules are injected into the bloodstream and then activated by a beam of ultraviolet light. It only takes a few minutes of light beam therapy to actively attack the cancer cells. The top research scientist

(Colin Self) stated: "I would describe this development as the equivalent of ultra-specific magic bullets." This breakthrough in cancer treatment is significant to Silver Sol because, according to Penn State University Professor Roy, Silver Sol has been published to resonate at a frequency of 910 terahertz which falls in the same category of ultraviolet light frequency as the antitumor lights (Curr. Science Invest, 2007).

It has been shown that infectious agents are associated with causing solid tumors (Kaposi's sarcoma), blood-based cancers (Leukemia) and other forms of cancers such as cervical cancer, which is caused by the Human Papilloma Virus. (Townsend Letters for doctors, May 2006). As you can see, bacteria, viruses, mold and other infectious agents have been reported to cause cancers. Taken daily, Silver Sol can prevent cellular bacteria, viruses, and mold so that the single-cell abnormalities never go beyond a single cell.

This is important because once diagnosed, doctors often prescribe chemotherapy or radiation that can cause immune suppression. This suppression of normal immune function allows for multiple pathogens to seed or spread. In this situation Silver Sol may have the potential to play a dual role: either destroy the infectious agent that causes the cancer and/or destroy the pathogenic load arising from the immunocompromised patients (Townsend Letters for Doctors. May, 2006).

Doctor Rentz (Am Acad Environmental Medicine, 2003) reports that the following cancer-associated infections are susceptible to Silver Sol treatment: HIV (Bull Cancer, 2006), Kaposi's sarcoma (Eur. Neurology, 2002), Epstein Barr Virus (J. Biol Regul Homeost Agents, 2005), Respiratory syncytial virus (Pediatrics, 2005), Influenza, Parainfluenza, Fungemia (J Support Oncology, 2005), Rotavirus (Bone Marrow transplant, 2005) Cytomegalovirus (Cancer, 25), and streptococcus pneumoniae (Medicine, 2005).

According to a NASA Technical report done at the University of Wisconsin, Silver Sol can be skillfully administered and due to its picoscaler diffusion capabilities will impregnate all collective atoms within each tumor cell or pathogenic cell with silver ions (Final technical report, University of Wisconsin, and NASA CR-114978, code 3, cat 04). This saturation potential supercharges silver's ability to displace the potassium-dependent glucose transport mechanism which is the exclusive means be which cancerous cells feed themselves, thereby selectively starving cancer cells without harming normal cells (Townsend Letter for Doctors, May, 2006).

Published cancer results include:

"We studied malignant fibrosarcoma cells (cancerous fibroblasts) and found that electrically injected silver suspended their runaway mitosis. (Becker, 1995).
Women with breast cancer (confirmed by biopsies), each received a single dose of Silver Sol at a concentration of 10 ppm. The 30 subjects were re-tested by biopsy at day 19 post injection, resulting in 100% normal tissue (Antelman, MS. 2000).

Canker Sores

Canker sores have a myriad of causes. Too much acid in the mouth is the number one cause. The tissue in the mouth gets destroyed by stomach acid, too many sugars, and bacterial or viral infections.

Silver Sol can help improve the issues quickly. Hold one ounce of Silver Sol liquid in your mouth for six minutes and then drink it. Repeat this process twice a day. Silver Sol gel can also be applied topically to the wound.

If the canker sore is a result of the herpes virus, the sooner you get the gel on the wound, the sooner you can stop the virus from replicating and getting worse. You should expect the wound to improve twice as fast with Silver Sol gel applied to the canker sore than if it were to run its course normally.

Candida
(see Yeast)

Cardiovascular Disease (Heart Disease)

Cardiovascular disease affects the heart, veins, arteries, and the circulation of blood and nutrients throughout the body. It is estimated that as much as 80 percent of all cardiovascular disease has its origin as a bacterial infection that originates in the mouth.

Cardiovascular disease can come from a bacterial infection like strep throat or a staph infection. By rinsing the mouth with Silver Sol liquid, you can kill the bacteria in the gums that lead to cardiovascular disease. This will also kill the bacteria that cause gum disease and bad breath.

Carpal Tunnel Syndrome

Carpal tunnel syndrome is characterized by painful swelling and inflammation in the joints. By drinking two teaspoons twice a day, or as needed, Silver Sol can help reduce pain and inflammation. Silver Sol gel can be applied topically to the joint if it is hot or red. Glucosamine, chondroitin sulfate, and essential fatty acids may also be used.

Cataracts

Cataracts cloud your vision, distort your view, and make it difficult to read and focus. Fortunately, the condition can be prevented and improved. Spray two or three drops of liquid Silver Sol directly in the eyes one to four times a day and drink two teaspoons twice a day for one week, or until the problem is remedied. Other products that can help include bilberry eyebright, lutein, and antioxidants.

You should expect to have an improvement in your eyesight very quickly, especially if you have very dry eyes or a bacterial or viral infection.

Cataracts that are very progressed are difficult to reverse, but the surface of the eye and the clarity of lens can be improved by using Silver Sol topically.

Cavities

Teeth are susceptible to cavities. Though the enamel is very hard, sugar and bacteria have the ability to eat away the enamel and cause cavities.

Rinsing your mouth with Silver Sol regularly will kill cavity-causing bacteria. Rinse your mouth for six minutes with one ounce of liquid silver two times a day. Then swallow two teaspoons to benefit your entire body. Coenzyme Q10 will also help improve gum health.

> I was on a trip with a man in his 30s. He started experiencing a lot of pain in a tooth and his gum line. The next day the mouth was more painful and it was very sensitive to water. It looked like he was starting to develop a cavity and an abscess was developing under his gum.
>
> He took a finger full of Silver Sol gel, placed it on his gums and rubbed it in. He also rinsed his mouth with Silver Sol liquid for six minutes. Before he had even finished, the pain was reduced significantly. He did not have to suffer for the next few days until he could get to a dentist. The abscess also reduced in size.
>
> In addition to brushing your teeth daily, I recommend brushing with Silver Sol gel once or twice a week. I also recommend a five-minute mouth rinse with a liquid gel once a week.

Chafing

Chafing occurs when skin rubs against skin or when another piece of clothing rubs against skin. The skin becomes reddened, a rash forms, and bleeding may occur. When applied to affected areas, Silver Sol gel will speed improvement and reduce pain.

A group of motorcyclists came in to see me after a long day of riding on the sand dunes. They all had chaffed areas from where their bottoms and their inner thighs had rubbed against their seats and gas tanks all day. Sand had gotten in their pants and chaffed them to the point that the skin was red and nearly bleeding.

They applied Silver Sol gel to these areas. Within five minutes, their pain was relieved and within two hours the redness was gone. By the next morning most of them had no problems at all. One rider had some scabbing, but it was pain free and there was no inflammation.

Children

Silver Sol is safe for use with children. Children require a smaller dose of liquid Silver Sol than adults. A 50-pound child, for instance, would take one-third the dosage of a 150-pound adult. Children will utilize the gel much more frequently, however, because they have poorer hygiene habits.

Silver Sol gel can be given to children one to four times a day, and they can drink Silver Sol liquid once or twice a day. For prevention, I recommend children take one-half teaspoon once or twice a day. This general dosage may be doubled during times of illness.

Cholesterol

Cholesterol is found among the fats in the arteries and veins. If too much fat accumulates, the blood can thicken and the fat can stick anywhere it is circulated. The liver is responsible for the fat levels in your blood and arteries. If the liver is not working optimally, enzymes are not produced correctly, fats are overproduced, and the liver gets clogged with cholesterol. The liver is then unable to detoxify the body and cholesterol levels continue to increase.

Cholesterol is not directly reduced by using Silver Sol. However, by combining it with a healthy diet, exercise, a reduction in fats, and plenty of exercise and water, it can help the liver function properly and keep cholesterol at a normal range. Take one teaspoon of Silver Sol morning and night. I would also recommend a liver cleanse with milk thistle.

Chicken Pox

Because chicken pox is a virus, Silver Sol can be very beneficial in neutralizing the problem. It can also help with the associated blistering and scarring. By applying the gel within four hours of the first outbreak, Silver Sol will help reduce the impact to the skin. Often the blisters will not completely arise and scarring will be lessened.

If you already have blisters, applying the gel topically one to four times a day will help conditions improve quickly. In addition, you should drink two teaspoons of Silver Sol twice a day. Chicken pox can return years later in the form of shingles. This dosage will also help with shingles.

Chlamydia

Chlamydia is a bacteria that is transferred by sexual contact. It destroys the tissues inside the vagina and can reoccur when the immune system is depressed. It is informally referred to as "clap."

Chlamydia is caused by bacteria inside the vagina and surrounding area. The symptoms of Chlamydia include pain, inflammation, rash and tissue damage.

- Drink two teaspoons of Silver Sol liquid twice a day for prevention.

- Use Silver Sol gel as a personal lubricant, on the male and female genitals, prior to sex. The gel is water-soluble and lubricates just like KY Jelly. Silver Sol gel will destroy sexually transmitted diseases like gonorrhea, syphilis, aids, Herpes simplex and chlamydia. You can also put gel on a condom to lubricate and destroy bacteria, viruses, and yeast that may be transferred during intercourse.

Chronic Fatigue Syndrome

Chronic fatigue syndrome has a number of different causes—viral, bacterial, hormonal, or parasitic. Important identifying factors include muscle and joint aches, stiffness, and fatigue. It can also affect hearing and eyesight.

Two tablespoons of Silver Sol can be taken two or three times a day for relief. Gel can be applied or sprayed on sore muscles once or twice a day as needed for aches and pains. Silver Sol liquid drops can be used in the eyes and ears as well.

Many people suffering from Epstein bar virus or mononucleosis have taken Silver Sol to help restore their energy. Additional products to help with chronic fatigue are coenzyme Q10 and freeform amino acids.

Circulation
(See also Cardiovascular Disease)

Circulation can be improved simply by taking the bacteria, viruses, and yeast out of the system. In addition to drinking two teaspoons of Silver Sol a day, use of vitamin E, dietary fiber, and antioxidant drinks can help.

Cleansing

Silver Sol helps cleanse the organs of excretion (colon, bladder, kidneys, etc.) by killing the bacteria, viruses and yeast that infect them. Remember it takes 6 minutes for the Silver Sol to completely kill these pathogens. In a cleansing situation Silver Sol will kill about 80% of the pathogen in as little as 15 seconds but if you keep the liquid or gel in contact with the pathogen for 6 minutes you will destroy the pathogen completely in almost all cases. Most people will use Silver Sol liquid 2 teaspoons twice a day. Apply the gel as needed to affected areas.

Colds

Colds are a virus. A cold gets in your nose and your sinuses and starts to duplicate there, producing a lot of mucus. Many will experience postnasal drip—mucus dripping down the back of the sinuses into the throat—when they go to bed. The mucus contains a virus or bacteria. When it reaches the back of the throat, it causes swelling and inflammation and can even spread into the ears.

Taking one tablespoon of Silver Sol three times a day, and spraying intranasally four or five times a day, will help reduce congestion and inflammation. Mouth rinse, eardrops, eye drops, nose drops, and throat spray can all be used as well.

Colitis, Irritable Bowel Syndrome, and Diverticulitis

Colitis is an inflamed colon. Irritable bowel syndrome is characterized by irritated and swollen bowels, and alternating constipation and diarrhea. Diverticulitis results from overstretched intestines that collect toxins—the body starts absorbing the toxins that should be passing out of the body and the toxins can get into the bloodstream.

By taking two teaspoons twice a day, Silver Sol will kill the yeast that causes these ailments. Herbs like catsclaw, digestive enzymes, and acidophilus will also help.

Colon
(See Enema)

Compress

Silver Sol gel taken from a refrigerator and put on a sterile gauze bandage can be used as a compress for bruises and wounds. It will help bring down a fever and will help compress sore or inflamed parts of the body. The cold temperature aids as a cold pack.

Congestion

Congestion—including nasal, lung, and upper respiratory—can stop you from breathing properly. Congestion leads to high production of mucus and can clog the nose, throat, sinuses, and lungs. If the congestion is caused by bacteria, it can last for months if the bacteria are not destroyed.

To remove congestion, spray Silver Sol into your nose one to four times a day and drink two teaspoons of the liquid twice a day. Inhaling silver 30 minutes a day will help lung congestion.

Congestion can create a poor sleep pattern and lead to decreased immune function. A hot, steamy shower will help you clean out your sinuses. Once the sinuses are clean, spray Silver Sol high into the nostrils. Rinse your mouth with Silver Sol as well, swallowing the solution when finished.

Constipation

Constipation has many causes, but foremost is lack of water. Bacterial or viral infections can create distress in your intestinal walls and decrease ability to absorb the proper amounts of water. Silver Sol can be of benefit when you drink one to two teaspoons twice a day. Acidophilus, fiber, and cleansing herbs will also help.

By keeping constipation at a minimum, you will keep toxins out of your bloodstream and neurotoxins out of your brain. You will cleanse all parts of your body and prevent the liver from becoming overloaded with detoxification work.

Conjunctivitis (Pink Eye)

Conjunctivitis results when bacteria build up on the surface of the eye. It can actually change the white of your eye, causing it to swell and turn pinkish red. If the inflammation is not reduced, the eyesight can be permanently damaged.

Silver Sol can help when you spray two or three drops of liquid Silver Sol directly into the eyes one to four times a day. Silver Sol gel can be placed directly into the eye where the gel will stay in place longer. Drink two teaspoons twice a day for one week or until the problem is remedied. This will usually remedy the problem within the first two to three days. Additional products that help are bilberry, eyebright, and lutein.

Crohn's Disease

Crohn's disease is an inflammation of irritable bowel syndrome. The main symptoms are abdominal pain, diarrhea (which may be bloody, though this may not be visible to the naked eye), constipation, vomiting, weight loss, or weight gain.

Though it is an infection, it is not clear if it is caused by bacteria, a virus, a parasite, or all three. By drinking four ounces of liquid Silver Sol the first day and two teaspoons of Silver Sol per day thereafter, you can destroy all three potential causes of the symptoms. Chrohn's disease is an autoimmune disease because the body attacks itself. For this reason silver is very good at destroying pathogens without inflaming the immune system.

In addition to Silver Sol liquid on a daily basis, you may want to consider adding acidophilus, cats claw, and coenzyme Q10.

Coughs and Croup

Coughs occur when your body is trying to rid mucus from the throat, lungs, and sinuses. Silver Sol can help with coughs and croup because it reduces inflammation and the bacteria or viruses that cause these coughs.

Silver Sol can help if you put three teaspoons in your mouth for six minutes. Allow a tiny amount of the liquid silver to trickle down the back of your throat every 30 seconds, then swallow the remainder. By doing this twice a day you'll have a significant amount of liquid silver passing across the cough or the irritated tissues that cause the cough. You may also pump Silver Sol intranasally as needed to stop a sore throat, congestion, or postnasal drip.

In addition, you may want to try inhaling Silver Sol from a nebulizer 15 minutes twice a day. Herbal expectorants in the form of mulen, pan pain lean, and immune stimulants like Echinacea can help as well. A warm shower is also recommended.

Cuticles

For cuticle care, soak your fingers in Silver Sol liquid for 30 minutes or apply Silver Sol directly. For cracked, dry cuticles, cover the hands with rubber gloves after applying the silver to seal in moisture.

Cysts

Cysts are usually the result of bacteria that collects under the skin. It grows and produces puss or other kinds of toxins. Take two teaspoons of liquid Silver Sol twice a day and apply the gel topically four times a day.

Dandruff

Dandruff is usually caused by dry, flaky skin. It can also be aggravated by a fungal or a bacterial infection. Apply Silver Sol to the scalp, rub it in, and allow it to stand for 10 minutes. This will stop bacterial and fungal infection and keep the scalp moist, reducing flaking.

Dengue Fever

Dengue Fever is an acute febrile disease found in the tropics and Africa. It is caused by four closely related viruses. Silver Sol can help when inhaled from a nebulizer 30 minutes a day and by drinking two teaspoons twice a day.

Unfortunately, Dengue fever can often get into parts of the body the silver has difficulty reaching. If this happens, increase the dosage to one teaspoon six times a day. If this doesn't work after two days, drink one full ounce and then return to the original dosage.

Depression

Depression can occur for a lot of different reasons, including biochemical and hormonal imbalances. A sedentary lifestyle can also lead to depression.

When a person has a depressed system, their chemistry needs to get back into balance. This isn't always easy. It requires a healthy diet and exercise. It has been found that people exercising 90 minutes a week over the course of eight weeks were able to control depression better than by taking antidepressant pharmaceutical drugs.

Bacterial and viral infections can have an effect on depression as well. Drinking one teaspoon of Silver Sol twice daily can keep these infections under control. St. John's Wort can help with mild to moderate depression and coenzyme Q10 can help with energy. A digestive parasite cleanse combined with Silver Sol can also improve depression by taking some of the toxins out of the intestinal system. Liquid Silver Sol can be taken one to two teaspoons one to three times a day.

Dermal Renewal

The dermis is a layer of the skin. The top layer of skin is basically dead. When we wash the skin the top layer flakes off. Deeper in the dermis, there is a continuous growth of new cells, producing new layers of healthy skin and tissues.

To help with dermal renewal, apply Silver Sol gel to skin anywhere on the body and then cover it with a plastic wrap. This keeps the gel from evaporating and allows it to penetrate deeper dermal layers of the skin. In addition, drink one teaspoon of liquid Silver Sol twice a day.

Detox Bath

Sometimes people want to rinse everything off their body—bacteria, viruses, mold, chemical substances, pollution, etc. To create a detox bath, fill your bathtub with warm water, pour in four ounces of liquid Silver Sol, and bathe for 20 minutes. This will allow you to wash every orifice of your body and all of your skin. Apply Silver Sol gel to your body after you get out, while the skin is still moist.

Diabetes

Diabetes is a problem associated with the islets of Langerhans cells in the pancreas. When these islets cells don't function properly, insulin is not produced and blood sugar gets out of balance. Those with no function in the islet of Langerhans or total pancreatic failure have Type-I diabetes. In Type-II diabetes (adult onset diabetes), the islets of Langerhans cells have partial or damaged function.

The damage to the pancreas can be caused by bacterial and viral infections. Drinking two teaspoons of Silver Sol twice daily can help fight these infections. Amino acids, coenzyme Q10, exercise, and healthy diet (with little to no refined sugars) will be beneficial.

Silver Sol does not cure diabetes; it helps prevent damage to the pancreas before diabetes sets in. Silver Sol gel can improve diabetic ulcers and wounds and is especially beneficial for foot wounds, venous stasis, ulcers, hemorrhoids, and varicose veins. Use the Silver Sol gel one to four times a day to keep these ulcers moist so they can improve more quickly.

Diarrhea and Dysentery

Diarrhea can be caused by a bacteria or virus. Dysentery is a bacterial infection. By taking a teaspoon of Silver Sol in the morning and at night, you can prevent these infections.

If you already have diarrhea or dysentery, you should swallow two teaspoons every hour for the first eight hours. The Silver Sol will help in as little as four hours. Complete improvement may take up to two days. Acidophilus can also be used.

> I experienced food poisoning and diarrhea after eating airplane food. I drank one ounce of Silver Sol every hour for the first two hours. My diarrhea stopped and I didn't have any further serious problems. This relief was very important because I had to continue traveling on the plane.

Diaper Rash

When babies wear diapers their skin can be in contact with urine for long periods of time. This warm, moist area of the skin will allow bacteria and fungus to grow very quickly. The skin becomes red and can even crack or bleed. By applying Silver Sol gel to the diaper rash you will be able to kill the cause of the diaper rash in the first two hours. The redness and pain can be remedied in as little as five minutes in mild cases.

To prevent diaper rash, you can spray a thin layer of Silver Sol on the inside of the diaper and then allow it to stand for about two minutes. This approach can also be used in children's socks to prevent athlete's foot.

Digestive System

Some common digestive system problems include excessive gas, diarrhea, yeast infections, or stabbing pains associated with a bacterial infection or food poisoning. Silver Sol liquid can help with each of these conditions. Drink two teaspoons every hour for about eight hours to help your digestive system. For daily prevention, drink one teaspoon twice a day.

Diverticulitis and Diverticulosis
(See Colitis)

Dry Skin

Dry skin occurs because we don't have enough fluids, oils, or essential fatty acids in our skin. It can also be caused by a bacterial infection, lack of exercise, or poor diet. Dry skin can lead to cracking, which allows infections to get into your system.

Silver Sol liquid and gel can be used to protect dry skin from infections. It should be applied to the dry skin one to four times a day. Silver Sol liquid can be taken one teaspoon twice a day. Aloe vera, amino acids, vitamin E or flax oil supplements can also be used.

Ear Drops
(See Ear Infections)

Ear Infections

Ear infections are a serious problem. In fact, Centers for Disease Control has requested that physicians no longer prescribe antibiotics for ear infections. The antibiotics make the problem worse by making the bacteria more resistant. We now have bacteria that we can't kill with antibiotics.

An ear infection can be a result of bacteria that gets in the inner ear and duplicates itself, destroying healthy tissue along the way. This could possibly leave a person deaf.

These bacteria can be destroyed by Silver Sol liquid after just five minutes of contact. Use a dropper to place five drops into the ear canal while the ear is pointed towards the roof. Keep the ear tilted up for 12 minutes. This will allow the Silver Sol liquid to get as far down behind the ear as possible. Repeat this process in each ear every 12 hours. You will also want to drink two teaspoons of liquid Silver Sol twice daily and take vitamin C.

While in a foreign country, I met a woman who had an ongoing ear infection. The infection had reached her inner ear and she was experiencing vertigo. She couldn't walk or move her head without losing her balance or becoming nauseated.

We put Silver Sol in her ear. She began to hear popping noises and felt the infection leaving her ear. After 10 minutes, we put the silver in her other ear. Twenty minutes later she was able to stand. The vertigo was gone. She continued to use Silver Sol as ear drops twice a day.

Endometriosis

Endometriosis is a condition where endometrial tissue is present outside of the uterus, causing severe uterine and/or pelvic pain.

The main symptom of endometriosis is pain concentrated in the lower abdomen. It may localize to one side of the abdomen or radiate to the thighs and low back. There is usually painful menstruation (dysmenorrhea), with different types of pain depending on the person—sharp, throbbing, dull, nauseating, burning, or shooting pains. Endometriosis may be long or short term; it may precede menstruation by several days or accompany it, but it usually subsides as menstruation tapers off. Severe pain may coexist with excessively heavy blood loss. On rare occasions nausea, vomiting, diarrhea, headache, dizziness or disorientation may occur.

Prostaglandins are inflammatory compounds released during menstruation that cause the muscles of the uterus to contract. Sometimes, the uterus muscles constrict so much that the blood supply is compressed, reducing the delivery of blood to the sensitive tissues of the endometrium. The absence of blood flow to the endometrium causes pain and cramping as the tissues die from lack of blood. The uterus begins to contract in such a strong manner that the dead tissues are squeezed out of the uterus and through the cervix and vagina. This temporary oxygen deprivation in the uterus is responsible for the cramps and pain. Silver makes dramatic improvements in wound healing and pain management inside the uterus. It also reduces inflammation, which can help reduce the cause of this painful disease.

- Swallow two teaspoons of Silver Sol liquid twice a day for prevention and treatment.
- Apply Silver Sol gel topically to affected area 2-5 times a day for as long as needed. You can also apply the gel to a tampon and insert into the vagina for 90 minutes a day. In this way the gel will stay in contact with wounds in the vagina.
- You can also create a Silver Sol douche. Use three ounces of Silver Sol liquid and mix it with three ounces of distilled water. Pump the solution into the vaginal cavity and hold for ten minutes, then release. This should be done once a day, for five days, or until symptoms are gone.
- There are optional uses of Silver Sol. Pour four ounces of Silver Sol liquid into a full tub of warm water. Soak and relax, flushing the silver water into the vaginal cavity. Twenty-five minutes is average for a muscle relaxing vaginal flush in the tub.

Enema

If you choose to use the silver as an enema it is most commonly used after the colonic or enema is completed and then a rinsing dose of 60 ml of Silver Sol liquid can be pumped into the colon. The gel can be used on the rectum to help prevent contamination or treat hemorrhoids.

Energy

When a person feels short on energy, their metabolism is usually in some form of disarray—often times the liver is damaged. By taking two teaspoons twice a day, Silver Sol has the ability to help restore proper function to the liver. This will help the liver secrete correct amounts of enzymes, detoxifying the body and allowing for more energy.

Enhances Antibiotic Function

Dr. Rustum Roy published studies that demonstrate the synergy of Silver Sol with antibiotics. Silver Sol makes some antibiotics ten times more effective at killing bacteria.

Antibiotics are rarely used for more than two weeks because they produce supergerms if utilized too long. Silver Sol does not produce this bacterial mutation because it destroys all the bacteria, resulting in a product that can be used daily without producing supergerms.

Epidemics, Pandemics

We are always at risk for an epidemic breakout, whether it is bacterial, viral, or parasitic. We've been warned that an influenza epidemic could kill as much as half of our population. Bird flu is also a real concern.

Liquid Silver Sol is one of the best tools in the event of an epidemic outbreak. The gel is necessary because most contagious diseases are transferred by hand contact. Silver Sol gel used on hands will help prevent as much as 70 percent of all contagious diseases.

One gallon of Silver Sol should be stored for each person in a home storage site. In addition to its anti-disease agent, it will help with water purification—four drops of Silver Sol will purify an eight ounce glass of water in less than two minutes.

To keep water safe for storage, pour approximately 16 ounces of Silver Sol liquid into a 50 gallon barrel of water, wait 10 minutes, and then seal it up. The water will stay safe for approximately four years.

Silver Sol can also be used topically, orally, intravaginally, intranasally, or inhaled. In the event of an epidemic, you may need any or all of these methods.

Epilepsy and Seizures

Epilepsy and seizures can by caused from a myriad of different situations. If it is bacterial or viral, Silver Sol can help. To help with seizures, drink one teaspoon twice daily.

In addition to Silver Sol liquid, put Silver Sol gel on your hands twice a day to help prevent contagious diseases from being transferred from your hand to your own body. Probiotics, phosphatidyl serine, coenzyme Q10 and minerals, B vitamins, and essential fatty acids can also help.

Epstein-Barr Virus

Epstein-Barr virus causes mononucleosis and chronic fatigue syndrome. Silver Sol has the ability to destroy viruses. Drink four ounces for two days, sipping every hour. Drink two ounces a day for the next five days. For maintenance, drink two tablespoons in the morning and at night. Use topically as needed.

If you have a uterine yeast infection at the same time, you can use Silver Sol as a douche, holding it for twelve minutes before releasing. If you need the gel for sore muscles, apply it topically and recognize that acidophilus, vitamins, minerals, and essential fatty acids with coenzyme Q10 may help.

Eyes

There are many problems that can develop within the eyes, both bacterial and viral. Most of them come from the outside, except for a few circulatory problems.

Spray two or three drops of silver liquid directly into the eyes one to four times a day and drink two teaspoons twice a day for one week, or until the problem is remedied. On a long-term basis, one teaspoon twice a day will suffice.

If you kill the bacteria and viruses on the surface of the eye you will reduce redness, inflammation and itchiness. Hopefully the proper tearing will be restored and you will have an eye that has a chance to heal itself fully.

After using Silver Sol, you should expect visible and noticeable differences in the first hour, with substantial improvements within two hours. Lutein, blueberry, and antioxidants also help.

Eye Wash Device

The proper use of an eye wash device can be very effective at delivering Silver Sol liquid into the eye. When there is a foreign object in the eye, Silver Sol liquid can be delivered using a specialized eye cap. This is also beneficial when used for eye infections, trauma or chronic conditions.

• Five drops of Silver Sol liquid can be used 1 to 5 times a day.

Eye Lift

Eyes seem to sag just from the effects of gravity. Skin holds itself together because of elasticity, which comes from elastin and collagen. By using Silver Sol, the cells of your skin start to pull together a little tighter, and a little faster. Take Silver Sol gel out of the refrigerator and apply while cold. The skin will tighten and firm for about two hours.

Face Lift

By applying refrigerated Silver Sol to your face, you will remove bacteria, viruses, and mold and see toning and tightening effects.

This also works on dark circles under the eyes, which are sometimes caused by toxins. Put a little gel under your eyes every morning and night and the silver will remove the dark color.

Facial Mask

Most facial masks only peel the dead skin cells off the surface of the face. Silver Sol can actually remove the toxins.

I recommend a powdered clay mix with added Silver Sol. When the clay is applied to the skin in liquid form, the silver will remove bacteria and firm and tighten the skin. The clay will remove oils and detoxify the skin, destroying the causes of acne and blemishes. Supplement by drinking one teaspoon of Silver Sol liquid twice a day.

Facial Peel

Some people use a facial peel to get down to the new and youthful layers of skin. These peels use harsh chemicals, basically burning the skin at the very top layer of its cells. By applying Silver Sol gel after a facial peel you'll experience quick improvements, better color, less pain and damage. You'll also get longer results with better cellular structure. One teaspoon of liquid Silver Sol should also be taken daily.

Facial Treatment

Silver Sol can be used as a facial treatment to help with regeneration of damaged cells, and wound management. It can also treat acne, infections, and premature aging. You will get the deepest Silver Sol penetration by washing the face with a mild soap, patting it dry, and then applying the gel to the skin while it is still moist. The gel can also be applied after steaming the face. This will open up the sweat glands and hair follicles and the gel will get deeper into the skin.

Applying the gel allows Silver Sol nano-particles to prevent infections by destroying bacteria, viruses, mold, and improve wound healing at the same time. It will also help prevent premature aging at the cellular level. You should also drink one teaspoon of liquid Silver Sol twice a day.

If you have sensitive skin, you will find that Silver Sol liquid and gel reduce inflammation, swelling, puffiness, and allergies.

Family Use

Families can utilize silver in countless ways around the home. It can be used to clean the shower or sink, to neutralize odors, or to freshen laundry. It is most beneficial, however, when used as a preventive agent. For a healthier family, each member should drink at least one teaspoon of Silver Sol once or twice a day. If there is an illness in the family, spray down the refrigerator, doorknobs, and bathrooms and increase the dosage to two teaspoons twice daily.

In the event of an epidemic like influenza or bird flu, there should be one gallon of silver stored in the home for each member of the family.

Fatigue
(see Chronic Fatigue Syndrome)

Fertility

Many women have a difficult time getting pregnant. Bacterial or viral infection could be the cause. Silver Sol should be taken orally, one teaspoon a day, to kill any infection inhibiting the ability to become fertile. Two ounces of Silver Sol may also be used as a douche, held intervaginally for 12 minutes and then released.

Men will want to drink one teaspoon twice a day and use Silver Sol gel as a personal lubricant to ensure bacteria is not transferred to the woman during intercourse. Amino acids, essential fatty acids, and antioxidants will also help fertility.

Fevers

Fevers are caused by bacteria, viruses, mold, foreign pathogens, and even sunburns. To break a fever, drink one teaspoon every hour (up to eight hours) until the fever breaks. Silver Sol gel can also be refrigerated and then applied topically to the forehead, temples, or anywhere else the fever is found.

If a fever does not break before it reaches 104 degrees, seek the care of a health care professional.

Fibromyalgia

Fibromyalgia is an autoimmune disorder with multiple symptoms. Though a single cause has not been identified, yeast seems to be a common factor. Yeast can leave the intestines and go into the brain. It can also be a neurotoxin, producing fermented fruits and vegetables in the intestines that can cause low dose alcohol toxicity.

By cleansing yeast out of the system, most fibromyalgia patients can control some of their symptoms. Yeast can be destroyed by drinking two tablespoons of Silver Sol two or three times a day. Gel or spray can be applied to sore muscles once or twice a day as needed for pain or aches. In addition to liver cleansing, vitamins, minerals, and freeform amino acids will all help with fibromyalgia.

Fingers

If you have sore or cracked fingers or cuticles—or a yeast infection under your fingernails or toenails—a Silver Sol soak can help. Soak your fingers in small dish of Silver Sol liquid for 15 minutes at a time.

The gel does not penetrate as deeply, but will stay in place throughout the day.

Follicle Detox

Shaving the face or legs can results in damaged hair follicles. Silver Sol gel can be used as a shaving gel to reduce bacteria, inflammation, swelling, and scarring.

Food Poisoning

Food poisoning typically includes symptoms such as nausea, vomiting, abdominal cramping, and diarrhea. It occurs suddenly (within 48 hours) after consuming a contaminated food or drink. It is usually caused by bacteria and viruses.

To fight food poisoning requires aggressive Silver Sol use, drinking about one ounce immediately, followed by two tablespoons every hour for the next eight hours. For prevention, drink one to three teaspoons a day. This can be especially helpful when traveling to a foreign country.

You can actually spray Silver Sol on food to kill the pathogens that cause food poisoning. After spraying, let it stand for two minutes before eating. E.coli and salmonella can also be killed by taking liquid Silver Sol.

Foot Bath

You should drink two tablespoons of Silver Sol before using a therapeutic footbath. These baths use electrolysis, sending a positive current through one end of an electrode and out through a negative electrode. Because silver is the best conductor of electricity, it will help in detoxifying the footbath.

You can also create your own footbath by placing Silver Sol in a bowl or tub, or by simply soaking washcloths and wrapping them around your feet.

Foot Odor

A very aggressive way to treat the feet is to soak them in warm water for 15 minutes. This will soften the dead skin on the surface, which can be scraped off with a loofah. Now the skin is ready and open for the gel to be applied to the entire foot. There are some seas salt scrubs that seem to help scrape the dead skin off with much more aggression. The EPA has approved the following claim for Silver Sol: "Silver Sol kills the bacteria that causes odor."

Foot Treatment Pack

Silver Sol gel and liquid can be very effective at killing fungus, yeast or bacteria that cause diseases of the foot. Specialized toe cots can be filled with Silver Sol gel and placed over the toe where the gel is pumped into and under the toenail. Slightly abrading (sanding) the toenail before applying the gel will allow better delivery of the gel.

- Before applying Silver Sol gel or liquid, first wash the foot and then remove the damaged, dead or diseased skin and nails. Do this by trimming the toenail, sanding the toenail and/or exfoliating the skin. Toes should be cotted twice a week until the toenail grows out healthy. Silver Sol gel can be applied to the foot twice a day after washing for use against bacteria and fungus.

Flu

Silver Sol liquid can prevent bird flu if taken daily. The animals that swallowed one teaspoon twice a day experienced a 100% increase in the ability to survive a fatal case of bird flu. The following is an abstract for this published study:

"Effect of Prophylactic Treatment with Silver Sol Solutions on an Avian Influenza A (H5N1) Virus Infection in Mice" August 30, 2007

Gordon Pedersen, Ph.D.   Colonel Robert Saum, Ph.D.
Robert Sidwell, Ph.D.   Keith Moeller
Colonel Alan Moloff, DO, MPH   William Moeller

Abstract

Female BALB/c mice were pre-treated with ASAP (Silver Sol) for seven days prior to being challenged with Avian Influenza (H5N1). The results were compared to control mice and Ribavirin treated mice to determine survival and prevention rates of Silver Sol on Avian Influenza (H5N1). Groups of 19 mice were treated by oral gavage (p.o.) with ASAP (Silver Sol 10 ppm) twice daily (every 12 h) for 7 days, then infected intranasally (i.n.) with an LD70 dose of influenza virus, then treated an additional 10 days. As controls, 35 mice were treated with water using the identical schedule as used for the ASAP materials and infected as above. Oxygen saturation (SaO2), necropsy for lung scores, and lung viral titers were tested to quantify ongoing tissue damage. As toxicity controls, 3 uninfected mice were treated in parallel with each test material and observed for signs of adverse effects for the next 21 days.

As a result of this experiment, 60% of the infected mice treated with Silver Sol (10 ppm) survived compared to the 30% in the placebo-treated controls. This is a 100% increase in the ability of mice to survive an H5N1 Avian Influenza challenge. Results of this study demonstrate suggested inhibitory and preventive effect on this virus infection as seen by either less animals dying in the treated groups than in the placebo-treated controls, delay in mean day to death, lessened SaO2 decline, modest inhibition of lung consolidation, and/or lessened virus titers in the lungs. In addition there was no sign or symptom of toxicity from the usage of Silver Sol in mice, even at extreme doses. If the human protection were similar to that found in mice, it could provide a significant advancement in the prevention of a potential pandemic event. The data from this study strongly suggests that daily oral use of Silver Sol will safely prevent avian influenza and improve survival rates in mice.

The person that wants to prevent the flu should take Silver Sol liquid two teaspoons twice a day, and inhale one tablespoon from an inhaler or nebulizer 30 minutes a day.

Gallbladder Disease

Gallbladder disease results from a breakdown in the digestive system. It can be very painful and can disrupt lives. Yeast and bacteria play a role in the disease. To fight these causes, drink two tablespoons of Silver Sol twice daily for two weeks. Reduce the dose to one tablespoon twice daily for two more weeks, and then maintain one teaspoon a day. Utilizing a proper gallbladder and digestive cleansing will also speed up recovery.

Gargle
(See Mouth Wash)

Gastritis and Gas

Gas can be produced from yeast and sugar mixing with fruits and vegetables in your intestines. It can also be produced directly from certain fruits, vegetables, and bacteria. Most people think that gas is produced by eating beans. In reality, a bacterium on the surface of the bean produces gas.

Silver Sol can help because it destroys bacteria that causes gas. If you have a gas outbreak—including painful air pressure in the intestines—take two teaspoons every hour for the first few hours.

In addition, you might want to try acidophilus and a digestive cleanse. Digestive enzymes can also be of assistance.

"Silver Sol is the most effective product I have ever worked with and is ranked number one by my patients. Not only is it the most effective, but it is the most researched technology on the market today." – Female gynecologist

Genital Herpes

Genital herpes is a virus affecting the genital area. Applying Silver Sol gel topically can help the outbreak improve more quickly. It should be placed on the genitals as soon as the outbreak occurs. In addition, drink two teaspoons of Silver Sol liquid twice a day. Daily silver use will also help prevent future outbreaks.

Geriatric/Elderly Use

People over age 50 can use Silver Sol as recommended. They can also take up to four times the normal recommendations if they have a serious or chronic illnesses, depressed immunity, anemia, or are around a large quantity of germs. The gel and liquid can be used in any orifice of the body.

Gingivitis

Silver Sol can be placed into the dental floss container and disinfect the floss that carves food off the tooth and gums. It also cuts into the gums and can cause infections, so pour two tablespoons of liquid Silver Sol into the dental floss container and use this disinfectant floss between your teeth.

Hand Disinfectant

Drink two teaspoons of Silver Sol twice a day, and apply Silver Sol gel to your hands one to four times a day, to help prevent problems associated with contagious diseases.

Hand Restoration

As we age, our hands are exposed to sunlight, cleansing agents, and drying agents. The skin gets wrinkled and damaged. By drinking one teaspoon of liquid Silver Sol twice a day, the silver will enter the red blood cells and work from the inside of the capillary system. Applying Silver Sol gel one to four times a day will benefit the topical layers of the skin.

Hay Fever
(see Allergies)

Headaches

Headaches can be caused by a number of different factors including bacteria, viruses, mold, allergens, and hormones. Because the brain does not contain pain receptors you cannot have a brain ache, but the veins and arteries that flow through your head can cause pressure and the circulatory system can feel pain.

By reducing the bacteria and viruses, Silver Sol will reduce the pain in the head. Drink two teaspoons twice a day and put gel on the temples twice daily. This will also kill the yeast, bacteria, and viruses that pass through the intestines into the bloodstream.

Healing Gel

In a study performed for the Singapore Department of Homeland Security, it was shown that Silver Sol liquid and gel improve wound healing by a factor of three times. This means wounds will close three times faster than normal. There will be three times less bacteria in the wound and inflammation is reduced by three times. This means it will help reduce scaring even those existing scars or stretch marks.

Silver Sol can be used topically as a healing gel on sunburns, scratches, scrapes, bites, or chemical burns. Because Silver Sol passes through the body unchanged, it produces no harmful metabolites and will help the healing process wherever the circulatory and capillary systems take it.

Healing gel should be used a minimum of once a day as a preventive agent and up to 12 times a day, as needed, to keep a wound moist. Silver Sol can be sprayed on, applied topically, or poured on as a liquid.

Hemorrhoids

Hemorrhoids are basically varicose veins at the rectum. These veins get irritated and swollen, causing a lot of pain. They get stretched out of shape and rupture with the passage of feces.

Silver Sol can help improve varicose veins by applying topically to the affected area twice a day or after every bowel movement. The gel can be used as a lubricant to help the stool move smoothly. It will also help inflamed tissues improve quickly. In addition, drink one teaspoon of liquid Silver Sol morning and night. A stool softener is also recommended.

> *I know a body builder who works out every day. He's very strong and muscular and also had hemorrhoids. They had become so bad that the doctors wanted to do surgery to remedy the problem.*
>
> *He decided to try silver. He applied the gel every day and after every bowel movement. He saw improvement the very first week. By two weeks, he was no longer waiting to have surgery. Now, a year-and-a-half later, the hemorrhoids are completely healed.*

Heart Disease
(See Cardiovascular Disease)

Hepatitis

Hepatitis is an inflammation of the liver that destroys its function and can be cause by viruses or bacteria. It is very difficult to treat but Silver Sol can be used in high doses to be beneficial. Silver Sol liquid can be swallowed 4 ounces a day for the first two weeks, and then swallowed two tablespoons twice a day for the next 3.5 months. This is a four-month attack on hepatitis. Gel can be used anywhere there might be contamination or transfer of germs.

Several successful subjects have used the drugs interferon and ribavirin at their lowest prescribed doses in combination with this protocol of Silver Sol. The liver numbers were reduced to near normal in one month and back to normal in two months and symptom-free in four months.

Herpes virus

Herpes viruses can affect the skin or the nervous system. When a herpes virus infects the inside or outside of the vagina, blisters and pain result.

The symptoms of the Herpes virus typically include water blisters inside and outside the vagina. These can be extremely painful depending on the severity of the lesions.

- Silver Sol liquid. Swallow two teaspoons of Silver Sol liquid twice a day for prevention and treatment. Also, apply the gel topically to affected area 2-5 times a day for as long as needed. Silver Sol gel can also be applied to a tampon and inserted into vagina for 90 minutes a day so the gel can stay in contact with germs in the vagina.

- To create a Silver Sol douche, use three ounces of Silver Sol liquid mixed with three ounces of distilled water. Pump the solution into the vaginal cavity and hold for ten minutes, then release. This should be done once a day, for five days, or until symptoms are gone.

- Take at least 8 billion active culture probiotic daily. Reduce dietary sugar and carbohydrates. And take large quantities of antioxidants daily. This will help neutralize and clear free radicals produced by pathogens.

Silver Sol can destroy the virus that causes infections in under six minutes. This means Silver Sol needs to stays in contact with the pathogen for at least six minutes. Most women feel noticeably better in one day and may return to normal in as little as two to five days.

High Blood Pressure

High blood pressure can be caused by hormones, blood or water volume, a change in biochemistry, a brain problem, or various other problems.

Silver Sol can reduce high blood pressure by helping the liver function normally and produce proper enzymes and cholesterol. Silver Sol can be taken in a liquid form, drinking two teaspoons twice a day. Dietary fiber should also be used.

Household Disinfectant

Silver Sol can be used as a disinfectant by spraying it on household items—toys, dishes, phones, purses, bathtubs, sinks, doorknobs, and so forth. After spraying items, let the solution stand for 10 minutes before wiping off. This will kill the bacteria throughout your home. Silver Sol gel can also be used, offering four hours of disinfectant power.

You may also want to spray the solution on your carpets, sheets and washcloths, or pour one ounce in the washing machine as you do the laundry. Put it in your disposal to help disinfect the bacteria and mold and control odors.

Silver Sol can be sprayed directly on vegetables or meats to help control E. coli and salmonella poisoning. It can also be used to disinfect jewelry or the baby's bed.

Human Papilloma Virus (HPV)

This is a viral infection usually afflicting the cervix. It destroys the cellular structure of the cells and can damage the DNA, causing cancer of the cervix.

Most of the time there are no symptoms of HPV infection. The only way to know if you have HPV is to have lab tests performed by a doctor. No real treatment is given until the tissues damaged by the virus have become cancerous. At this point surgery is performed. If a woman uses Silver Sol liquid (douche) and gel on a tampon she can destroy the virus that causes the abnormal cells, possibly preventing the cause of the cancer.

- Swallow two teaspoons of Silver Sol liquid twice a day for prevention and treatment.

- Apply Silver Sol gel to a tampon and insert into vagina for 90 minutes a day so the gel can stay in contact with germs in the vagina.

- To create a Silver Sol douche, use three ounces of Silver Sol liquid mixed with three ounces of distilled water. Pump the solution into the vaginal cavity and hold for ten minutes, then release. This should be done once a day, for five days, or until symptoms are gone.

- Take at least 8 billion active culture probiotic daily. Reduce dietary sugar and carbohydrates. And take large quantities of antioxidants daily. This will help neutralize and clear free radicals produced by pathogens.

Silver Sol can destroy the virus that causes HPV in under six minutes. Most women feel noticeably better in one day and may return to normal in as little as two to five days.

> *"I used Silver Sol on Human Papillomavirus (HPV) warts. The patient had an outbreak around the rectum. Placed gel on warts for ten days. There was a 90 percent reduction of the HPV warts in ten days." – from a certified Urologist*

Hypertension
(See High Blood Pressure)

Hypoglycemia

Hypoglycemia means low blood sugar. Hypoglycemic individuals experience spikes and drops in blood sugar, especially when eating something sugary. This fluctuation makes a person very susceptible to bacterial disease and makes healing difficult. Improvements can be experienced by taking two teaspoons of Silver Sol twice a day and applying gel directly to wounds.

Immune Modulator

In HIV patients Silver Sol liquid was used 1 oz twice a day for four months and improved immune function an average of 40%. This means in an autoimmune and virus induced compromise, the Silver Sol liquid can improve the cellular number and reduced all symptoms of the AIDS patients. In normal people the improvement is less but the over protection is greater.

Impetigo

Impetigo is a bacterial infection of the skin that shows up as blisters usually around the mouth. For prevention, drink one teaspoon of Silver Sol twice a day. If you already are suffering from impetigo, drink two teaspoons twice a day and, more importantly, apply the gel topically one to four times a day. By keeping impetigo moist with Silver Sol gel, it will spread less and improve much quicker. Since impetigo is contagious you will want to apply the Silver Sol gel to your hands as well in order to prevent contaminating yourself or others.

"The first round of bottles has been used in about 85 patients consisting of adults and children, with great success for skin ulcers, fungus on the skin and nails, throat infections, tonsillitis, chicken pox and other skin bumps, badly infected cuts and wounds, ear infections, asthma and respiratory infections, and herpes. Everyone is very pleased, especially with the lack of side effects that strong antibiotics would have had. So the question is how can we get some more Silver Sol quickly!"

—from a letter from a ministry in Nicaragua that uses Silver Sol

Immune Support

Silver Sol helps modulate immune response but its real benefit is that there are fewer germs afflicting the immune system. Since the immune system can be overworked by our germ-filled environment, it must prioritize its efforts. This means the immune system fights germs first, then builds and rebuilds tissue if it has the capacity to do so. By reducing the ever-present germ burden on an overworked immune system, the ability to heal increases significantly. People with autoimmune diseases can be confident in using Silver Sol on the skin and inside the body because it reduces inflammation, activates stem cells, and promotes normal healing.

Infants Health

Babies can use a lower dose of Silver Sol—half a normal adult dosage. The liquid and gel can be used on or in any orifice of the body. Infants 0-6 months old would take one-half teaspoon (of liquid silver) twice a day. Babies 6 months and older and weighing up to 75 pounds would take a dose of one teaspoon twice a day. Children over 75 pounds would take a normal adult dose of two teaspoons twice a day.

Infections, Bacterial
(See Anti-Bacterial)

Infections, Viral
(See Anti-Viral)

Infectious Disease

Any time you are exposed to an infectious disease you are at risk of having significant cellular, systemic, or tissue damage. It can also be fatal. To prevent the spread of infectious disease, apply Silver Sol gel to your hands every four hours. This will keep pathogens from getting on your face or in your eyes, and will prevent the transfer of disease to others.

Inflammation and Swelling

Inflammation is almost always caused by bacteria, viruses, parasites, or mold. Silver Sol can fight these causes. Drink two teaspoons twice daily and apply the gel to inflamed areas as needed. Sometimes an inflammatory response is found around an open wound like an MRSA or staph infection. In this case, spray the gel on the affected area twice daily.

Influenza
(See Flu)

Inhaled Silver Sol

Silver Sol can be inhaled from a nebulizer (a nebulizer can be obtained at a medical supply store). The nebulizer creates a mist that you can inhale through a tube. This approach is very effective against bacteria, virus, and mold problems in the lungs and respiratory tract. Silver Sol should be inhaled 30 minutes a day—15 minutes in the morning and evening, or 30 minutes at once. The liquid mist can destroy infections such as tuberculosis and pneumonia.

Intestinal Detox
Silver Sol can help with intestinal detoxification. It can destroy yeast, bacterial, or viral infections. One hour after using a slippery elm product, cascara sagrada, laxative, or any other intestinal cleanse, use Silver Sol to remedy any infections.

Intravenous Treatment (IV)
(See Cancer)

Irritable Bowel Syndrome
(See Colitis)

Itching and Scaling

Itching and scaling can occur for a lot of reasons—bacteria, viruses, fungi, and allergies are just some. Regardless of the cause, dry skin is always a factor. Silver Sol gel will reduce pain, inflammation, itching, and scaling. The gel can be applied to children and adults of any age. Silver Sol can also be used to remedy poison ivy.

Jock Itch

Many men suffer from jock itch, or red, inflamed skin. If you live in a warm, humid, or tropical climate, you may have a fungal or bacterial infection that grows in the warm, moist folds of the skin, including the groin. Simple application of the Silver Sol gel twice daily should keep it under control. For more aggressive cases, it can be used five times a day. In addition, one teaspoon of Silver Sol liquid should be taken twice a day.

I went on a trip to Africa. I saw public advertisements all over the streets about treating fungal infections in the groin area. In Africa's warm, moist, tropical climate, this affects both men and women. People are making such extended use of gels, ointments, and antibiotics that their immune systems are being damaged.

Individuals who applied Silver Sol gel found relief from itching in five minutes, with the redness and inflammation leaving in two hours.

Joints
(See Arthritis)

Keratosis

Many people have precancerous legions from sun damage on their shoulders, chest, and face. It presents itself as dry, flaky skin spots or small, reddened, inflamed areas on the skin for years before it becomes a skin cancer.

Silver Sol gel can be applied topically once or twice a day, and one teaspoon of liquid silver can also be taken twice a day. I have seen a case of keratosis remedied in as little as two weeks. Treatment should generally be followed for at least two months.

Kidney Disease

Silver Sol passes through the body totally unchanged and does not produce harmful metabolites. It will pass through the intestines, bloodstream, kidneys and urine, producing anti-bacterial and anti-viral effects.

To help kidney disease, drink two teaspoons four times a day. (A smaller person will use one teaspoon four times a day.) This high dosage is necessary because it needs to pass through the kidney on a regular basis. As it passes through, it will disinfect and help bring the kidney infection under control in as little as 12 hours.

Lacerations

Taking two teaspoons twice daily of Silver Sol combined with a gel application four times daily can result in rapid recoveries without infection. The following is a quote from the *Journal of Healing Outcomes* on a patient who used the gel and liquid Silver Sol on a serious laceration. The following is a conclusion of why the Silver Sol works so successfully:

The topical application of Silver Sol gel kills pathogens and helps protect the wound from becoming contaminated or infected which means that the inflammatory phase of wound healing received significant assistance possibly by reducing the need for macrophages, monocytes and fewer cytokines producing less inflammatory response hormones. The fact that there is less inflammation suggests that there is a significant reduction in the inflammatory phase of healing. Since the Silver Sol destroys bacteria, viruses and mold the wound was not infected thus reducing the need for phagocytosis, which reduces the immune cascade required for clotting and decontamination of the wound. The elimination of bacteria leaves the wound edges and margins clean and capable of optimal healing. In addition there is an increased ability to secrete stem cells, which will produce multi-potent cellular healing. This produces obstacle free wound healing making a cleaner healing scar. This can be seen in the fact that the wound was closed and stitches removed by day three where the wound presented a very low amount of inflammation, with no bacterial contamination. This could help explain why there is very little scarring. This could also be due to the fact that with less inflammation, there is less need for the platelets to produce histamine, cytokines and prostaglandins, which results in less overall swelling which means the wound can heal faster due to the fact that there are less factors competing with collagen. This reduced inflammation results in more collagen filling the fibrin - fibronectin matrix producing less tension, better bridging to migrate across the wound and less constriction (fibrotic scarring of the wound). In addition the gel provides a wound that is moist promoting the migration of polymorphonuclear cells stretching across the wound, which can lay the foundation of a healthy uncomplicated wound. In addition it appears that stem cell activation (as published in Nexus 2008), could be responsible for the rapid adhesion of the laceration and assist in the removal of the scab and reduction of the scarring. This could occur because the endothelialization had less opposition from bacteria, mold and inflammation. It appears that stem cells had activated and mobilized angiogenesis from the healthy blood vessels as evidenced by the pink coloration of the tissues immediately surrounding the suture lines which indicate that stem cell activated angiogenesis had taken place with remarkable results probably due to the fact that there was no bacterial infection nor any contamination and its associative inflammation.

In short the Silver Sol appears to play a significant role to decontaminate, prevent infection and stimulate stem cells resulting in improved wound healing characterized by reduced inflammation, improved angiogenesis, more efficient phagocytosis and reduced scarring.

Since there is less need for polymorphonulclear cells there will be less helper T cells secreteting cytokines that cause the multiplication of inflammatory factors. This means there is less clean-up of inflammation and the wound in general. In addition there will be better stem cell production from the healthy fringes of the blood vessels, better collagen production and improved circulation due to the fact that vasodilation and blood vessel permeability will be normalized sooner in an uninfected and less inflamed wound. All of these parameters seem to have one thing in common; Silver Sol has antimicrobial abilities that help reduce infection, and inflammation resulting in better healing. Since inflammation lasts as long as there is debris or infection in the wound, it can be said that Silver Sol can help remove the cause of a significant amount of infection and inflammation. This results in improved healing outcomes by reducing the pathogenic burden on the immune system allowing optimal restorative and regenerative immune functions.

Leukemia

Leukemia is a cancer of the blood or bone marrow and is characterized by an abnormal proliferation of blood cells, usually white blood cells. Silver Sol can help with leukemia by drinking four ounces for two days, sipping it every hour. Drink two ounces a day for the next five days. Drink two tablespoons in the morning and at night for maintenance. Remember milk thistle to help cleanse the liver, and pa pa and antioxidants to help cleanse the bloodstream.

Leprosy

Leprosy is bacteria that have become resistant to antibiotics. In biblical times, it was the worst contagious disease in existence. Those suffering from it were quarantined to leper colonies. It may surprise you to know that there are still leper colonies today in Hawaii.

Silver Sol can destroy leprosy. By drinking two teaspoons two to three times a day and applying Silver Sol gel topically three times a day, you can fight even the most serious leprosy wounds. Lepers have been able to bring their disease under control within two days using Silver Sol.

Leichmaniasis

Leichmaniasis is a parasitic infection. It shows up just under the skin as a purple rash and raises welts and boil-like symptoms all over the body. Soldiers in Afghanistan have been suffering from this infection and it has been very difficult to remedy.

The army hospital at William Beaumont Army Medical Hospital conducted a study on leichmaniasis, using Silver Sol liquid and gel. They found that the parasite could be destroyed by drinking two teaspoons two to three times a day. The gel should also be applied two to four times as needed. You can expect to see a benefit over the course of eight weeks.

Lips

Many people suffer from chapped lips, the herpes virus (cold sores), or the lead in their lipstick. Placing Silver Sol gel on the lips every night will help to improve the lips and help to prevent damage. In addition, drink one teaspoon of Silver Sol liquid twice a day.

Lip Balm

It is easy to create your own silver lip balm. By adding a little bit of heat, you can melt your preferred lip balm. Add a small amount of liquid silver and then let the balm re-thicken. This will allow you to enjoy the benefits of silver each time you moisten your lips.

Liver Disease (see also Hepatitis)

The liver is one of the most important organs of the body. It detoxifies the blood and secretes over 4,000 enzymes. When the liver is inflamed, like in the case of hepatitis, it won't secrete as many enzymes and the blood will not be purified as quickly.

Silver Sol can destroy the bacteria and viruses that harm the liver. By restoring proper liver function, all systems of the body are benefited, and overall wellness is increased. For these results, drink two tablespoons of Silver Sol twice daily. For severe cases of hepatitis, this amount should be doubled.

Lung Disease

Our lungs can be damaged by cigarette smoke, toxins, and bacterial or viral infections. Silver Sol has been shown to destroy tuberculosis in laboratory testing. The lungs can be helped from both the inside and outside by drinking two teaspoons of Silver Sol daily and inhaling from a nebulizer 15 minutes twice a day.

Silver Sol can also be put in a humidifier and used while sleeping at night. For serious conditions, Silver Sol may also be taken intravenously.

Lupus

Lupus is an autoimmune disease that can affect various parts of the body, including the skin, joints, heart, lungs, blood, kidneys, and brain. Because it is an autoimmune disease, you can't use major immune stimulation products. Silver Sol can be used to the kill bacteria, viruses, mold, and parasites that may be the cause of the lupus. It will do this without making the lupus symptoms worse.

Silver Sol can be of benefit when you drink one teaspoon three times a day. It can also be applied topically to facial rashes commonly caused by lupus. In addition, you can use acidophilus, antioxidants, coenzyme Q10, and an intestinal cleanse.

Lyme Disease

Lyme disease is caused by the bacteria Borrelia burgdorferi. It is primarily transmitted to humans by the bite of infected ticks belonging to a few species of the genus Ixodes ("hard ticks"). Lyme disease can also come from infected mice, horses, dogs, cattle, birds and rodents. It is the most common vector-borne disease in the United States.

Clinical manifestations of Lyme disease are divided into three stages: 1. Flu-like symptoms and a bulls-eye type of skin rash (erythema migrans). 2. Weeks or months later, Bells palsy or meningitis-type of neurologic symptoms develop. 3. Months to years later, arthritis develops. Symptoms get progressively worse if the cause of the disease is not eliminated.

Physicians usually prescribe antibiotics such as doxycycline, ceftriaxone, or amoxicillin. These seem to be fairly effective against Lyme disease if given within the first two weeks of infection, but the efficacy may diminish over time due to the progressive nature of the disease.

Ticks feed once during each of their three stages of life: larval ticks feed in late summer, nymphs in the following spring, and adults during the fall. Most human infections occur during the summer months. Under laboratory conditions the tick was required to feed for 24-36 hours or longer to transmit infections. This means that a human must have the infected tick feeding on them for two days in order to get infected. So the first line of defense against Lyme disease is to spread Silver Sol gel on high-risk areas of the skin on a daily basis. This daily surveillance should prevent the tick from infecting the skin for a 36-hour period.

- If you think you have been bitten by a tick within the past two weeks, drink two ounces of liquid Silver Sol a day and apply gel to the bite four times a day for two weeks.

- If you have Lyme disease, drink two ounces of Silver Sol liquid twice a day and apply gel to affected or sore areas twice a day. Continue this for three months, then reduce the dose by half for a month and return to full dose for a month and continue as long as needed. The reason to alternate high and low doses is because the bacterium drills down into muscle and hide from treatment, but rises up out of the muscle when not attacked so a high dose can be more effective a month later. Note: Some people who have a difficult case of Lyme disease may want to drink eight ounces of Silver Sol at one time to initiate this treatment.

For prevention of Lyme disease, drink two teaspoons of Silver Sol liquid twice a day and apply Silver Sol gel twice a day.

Lymphatics

Lymphatics are used to cleanse the lymph system. The lymph system is parallel to the circulatory system in that it has glands in all the major circulatory areas. But the lymph system does not have a heart or a pump attached to it. Lymph flow is controlled by the movement of the body.

Since the lymph is only circulated when the body moves, it is essential to walk, move your arms, stretch, and exercise to make your lymph system circulate out all of the toxins. A sore throat, for example, occurs when the lymph glands gather bacteria that are being circulated through the lymph, into the circulatory system, and out of the body.

To help the lymph system do its job of getting the toxins and bacteria out of the body, drink two teaspoons of Silver Sol twice a day and apply the gel to affected areas twice a day.

Malaria

Swallow two ounces of liquid Silver Sol every day for two weeks and apply Silver Sol gel four times a day to wounds (if necessary). For prevention swallow two teaspoons twice a day and apply gel as needed.

I traveled to Ghana, where we gave liquid Silver Sol to children with malaria. We saw even the most severe cases remedied in five days. These children continued to follow the treatment for 10 days.

I saw one two-year-old child who was literally hours away from death, suffering from ear and throat infections and fever associated with malaria. Within four days of using silver he was completely healthy.

Makeup Base

Silver Sol can be used in addition to, or in place of, makeup base. After you wash your face, apply a thin layer of Silver Sol gel. Wait two minutes for it to dry and then apply your base. This will give you protection against acne, blemishes, and infections from mold, bacteria, and viruses.

Some women use the Silver Sol gel as their base and natural coloring. This approach can replace damaging makeup and allergenic topic cleansing, as it washes clean with water.

Makeup Irritation

When people put on makeup everyday it often begins to irritate their skin. The skin may become red and itchy and rashes can form. To neutralize this problem, apply Silver Sol gel and drink Silver Sol liquid on a daily basis.

One teaspoon of Silver Sol liquid should be taken twice daily. In addition, when the makeup is removed, soak a cotton ball with silver and wipe the face clean. This will neutralize pathogens that may aggravate or irritate the skin. It will also help with pain, redness, and skin regeneration.

To add another layer of protection, Silver Sol should also be applied at night before bed. Hypoallergenic makeup will also prevent irritation problems.

Massage Therapists and Other Health Care Professionals (For Protection)

Massage therapists have one great enemy, infection. The patients bring infections on their skin in the form of acne, rashes, staph, blisters, streptococcus, and yeast. These are highly contagious and can be spread from patient to therapist. Some of the infectious agents like MRSA (methicillin-resistant Staphylococcus aureus) can be transferred by touch and can infect the patient, therapist and surrounding environment, leaving everyone who enters the room at risk of a potentially fatal infection. There are hundreds of therapists that have contacted MRSA from their patients. I recommend Silver Sol for massage therapists and all other medical professionals who come in contact with skin. They should use it for self-protection as well as protection for their patients.

- Apply Silver Sol gel to any at-risk regions of the skin, nose, eyes, face or other exposed skin areas as often as needed (usually 1-10 times a day). Drink two teaspoons of Silver Sol liquid twice a day.

Memory Enhancement

Memory can be negatively impacted by bacteria-caused inflammation. Silver Sol can help reduce the inflammation by drinking two teaspoons twice a day. By inhaling silver from a nebulizer, it can go straight to the brain. Inhale 15 minutes a day for memory enhancement and 30 minutes for infectious issues. Phosphatidylserine, coenzyme Q10, ginkobaloba, and B complex vitamins can help as well.

Menopause

Menopause is the complete shutting down of the female reproductive system. Silver Sol helps make hot flashes less significant by fighting bacterial, viral, or vaginal yeast infections. It also reduces the aches and pains associated with menopause. The liquid can be taken every day, one teaspoon twice a day, or as needed. The gel can be applied to any painful area of the body, including the breasts.

Migraine Headaches
(See Headaches)

Mold and Fungus

Fungus and mold grow in warm, moist, and sugared areas such as the intestines or vagina. Taking sugar out of your diet and using silver both topically and internally can treat these. Take two teaspoons of silver three times a day and apply it topically one to four times a day, if needed. This dosage should be continued for at least two weeks longer than symptoms are present.

You can expect to see a benefit within the first 30 minutes. It will take at least 10 minutes for the liquid to kill a fungal infection on the skin. Silver will work best when taken with complementary products such as probiotics, caprylic acid, anti yeast diets, essential fatty acids, and amino acids.

Silver can also be sprayed on household items. In about 10 minutes it will kill the fungus, bacteria, or viruses on your table, food, clothes, phone, refrigerator, or toilet.

Mononucleosis

Mononucleosis is an infection that produces flu-like symptoms. To relieve the symptoms, drink four ounces for two days, sipping every hour. Drink two ounces a day for the next five days. For maintenance, drink two tablespoons in the morning and at night. Use topically as needed.

Mouth Wash

Dental floss can be used in combination with the mouthwash. It will prevent infection if you pour 2 tablespoons of the liquid Silver Sol into the dental floss container and floss with silver soaked string.

Morgellons

Morgellons is a disease that presents itself in many ways, but all of them involve inflammation, swelling tissue damage and dry, flaky, pustulant skin rashes. Some believe it is caused by a parasite, and others think it is caused by a fungus. In either case the solution can be Silver Sol, which destroys bacteria, viruses and yeast.

- Apply the gel as often as needed to keep the skin moist because it seems to heal better when it is not dry and flaky. Drink two tablespoons of the liquid twice a day. In cases where the skin is extremely dry and flaky, a moisturizing product like aloe vera can be mixed with the Silver Sol to keep skin moist. Two parts aloe gel mixed with ten parts Silver Sol gel makes a product that will help dramatically. Note: A moist wound is important to minimize the rash but a wound that is too wet will become macerated.

MRSA and Staph

MRSA (Methycillin resistant Staphylococcus aureus) is a resistant variation of the common bacterium Staphylococcus aureus. The organism is resistant to a significant group of antibiotics called the beta lactase, which includes penicillins. MRSA is approaching pandemic levels. There is an immediate need for a substance like Silver Sol in controlling this potentially fatal disease. According to the Journal of the American Medical Association (JAMA Oct. 2007), MRSA was responsible for 94,360 serious infections and associated with 18,650 hospital–stay related deaths in the United States in 2005. The statistics suggest that MRSA infections are responsible for more deaths in the U.S. each year than AIDS.

Symptoms of MRSA usually manifest as a patch of small pus surrounded by redness and swelling. It may resemble a pimple, spider bite, or boil and may not be accompanied by a fever. The bumps become larger and spread and these larger pus-filled boils can develop deep into the tissue. Most cases infect the skin; a minority of these infections can invade vital organs and cause sepsis, toxic shock syndrome, flesh eating (necrotizing) and pneumonia.

- Drink two tablespoons of Silver Sol liquid three times a day. This is triple times the normal dose and will work nicely if taken as needed until symptoms subside.

- Apply Silver Sol gel to the affected area and surrounding tissue 2-6 times a day.

Currently Silver Sol is the only prophylactic that has activity against MRSA. It can be used for prevention as well as treatment of MRSA. It is important to note that daily use of Silver Sol does not produce resistant strains of MRSA.

> *"My son was on the wrestling team in high school. He got an MRSA infection from the wrestling mat, they say. He missed school for a month and could not wrestle because he had a contagious rash. It was eating his flesh. The antibiotics helped but could not get rid of it. He started using Silver Sol—drinking two tablespoons twice a day and putting the gel on his rash twice a day. He got better in three weeks and is now wrestling again. The coach sprays the mat with Silver Sol every day and gave a tube of gel to every team member. I find that families are using it at home too."*

Multiple Sclerosis

Multiple sclerosis (MS) is an autoimmune condition in which the immune system attacks the central nervous system. It can be impacted dramatically by Silver Sol when you drink two tablespoons, three times a day and inhale Silver Sol 15 minutes a day.

By drinking liquid Silver Sol, the silver gets into circulation and can get to the base of the brain stem. By inhaling, it will reach the brain stem a bit quicker. This will prevent the secondary effects associated with multiple sclerosis. In addition, MS can be benefited by arginine, coenzyme Q10, B-complex vitamins, and lesafin.

Myocardial Infarction

Myocardial infarction (MI) is a condition where the heart often stops beating and is usually caused by the clogging of heart arteries. This usually begins with problems in the mouth and gums.

To kill the bacteria in the mouth, one ounce of liquid Silver Sol should be held in the mouth for six minutes and then swallowed. By doing this daily, you can destroy the bacteria that causes damage to the heart and heart valves.

Neck Firming Cream

When a person ages, the skin can stretch due to the loss of elastin and collagen. By applying Silver Sol topically to the neck, you will remove the fungus and bacteria that may reside in the dead skin cells or wrinkles of the neck. The wrinkles will stop growing deeper and you will have a more youthful-looking skin. In this way you'll have better skin texture. To achieve these benefits, put Silver Sol gel in the refrigerator, take it out, and apply while cold 1-4 times a day.

Nerves

Nerves transmit electrical and chemical energy, directing the movement of the body. Any inflammatory disease will inflame the tissues, which will put pressure on the nerves and send pain throughout the body. Silver Sol can reduce inflammation, pain, and pressure on the nerves.

Two teaspoons of liquid silver can be taken internally daily. Silver Sol gel can also be applied to the affected areas to help reduce inflammation and pain associated with nerves problems.

Night Cream

You might want to mix your toner or moisturizing cream with Silver Sol to produce an antibacterial toner or moisturizer. The moisturizer would require you to pour out 20% of the moisturizer and replace it with Silver Sol liquid. Shake well and use to prevent pathogens while moisturizing. The same percentages work for toners (20% Silver Sol liquid with 80% toner).

Nose and Sinuses

Nose and sinus congestion can stop you from breathing properly. Congestion leads to high production of mucus and can clog the nose, throat, sinuses, and lungs. If the congestion is caused by bacteria, it can last for months if is not destroyed.

By applying three or four sprays of liquid Silver Sol internasally, you will protect the nose and sinuses from developing a bacterial, viral, or fungal infection. This should be done two to four times a day. In addition, drink one teaspoon of Silver Sol twice a day. This will reduce sinusitis, colds, and other problems associated with nasal congestion.

Nose Drops

Using an intranasal sprayer or dropper, you can pump Silver Sol liquid into your sinuses. You can also tip your head back and use silver as nose drops. This allows the liquid to flow through your sinuses. You will feel it flow out on the back or your throat, where it will help detoxify the sinuses and throat.

Many people get recurring sore throats from postnasal drip, which is when mucus drips from the sinuses into the back of the throat. Nasal drops and nasal spray will help remedy postnasal drip and congestion.

Obesity

Silver Sol does not burn fat, thus it does not change obesity. Obesity compresses arteries, nerves, the stomach, and the overall amount of fats in the intestines. This causes circulatory, hormonal, and intestinal problems.

Drinking two teaspoons of Silver Sol twice a day and using it topically as needed can help with some of the problems associated with obesity.

The silver will destroy excess yeast in the intestines. It will also reduce scarring caused by stretch marks. Digestive and liver cleansing and milk thistle should be used in combination with the Silver Sol when targeting obesity.

Orifices

Silver Sol can be used in any orifice of the body—eyes, ears, nose, mouth, rectum, or vagina.

Osteoporosis

Osteoporosis is a disease of bone that leads to an increased risk of fracture. Though Silver Sol will not help with the thinning of the bone, it will help with wound healing by reducing the fungus, bacteria, and mold that may otherwise inhibit healing. Using calcium, magnesium, and vitamin D twice a day will also help.

Pain

Pain is a very important tool for diagnosing disease. Most people don't even think about checking themselves for an illness or getting treatment until they feel pain.

Silver Sol gel can be used topically to reduce mild and moderate pain. Drinking one teaspoon of liquid silver each day will also help. If the pain persists, you should visit the doctor to see if there is a problem. Using antioxidants and stretching will also reduce pain.

Pancreas

Pancreas problems cause blood sugar to get out of balance, leading to diabetes and depression. Pancreatitis is caused by a viral or bacterial infection, usually from bad food or water. Because pancreas issues can escalate quickly, it is important to take Silver Sol on a regular basis, drinking two teaspoons twice a day.

Parasites

The World Health Organization estimates that one in four people have a chronic parasitic infection of some kind. It may be in the intestines, under the skin, or in the lungs. Parasites can come from the food we eat, including pork and fish. Once they are inside our bodies, they lay eggs. The eggs hatch and take up residence in the body, and then the process is repeated. It is important to get rid of parasites permanently.

Silver Sol can help. It does not kill all parasites, but it does help in the intestines, in the blood, and with leichmaniasis. Silver Sol will need to be used for three months, as the lifecycle of each generation of parasites is about 45 days. During this time, drink two teaspoons twice a day. Black walnut hulls, digestive cleansing, and milk thistle will also help this process.

Parkinson's Disease

Parkinson's Disease is a degenerative disorder of the central nervous system that often impairs the sufferer's motor skills and speech, as well as other functions. Brain inflammation is also associated with the disease. By drinking Silver Sol two teaspoons twice daily and taking methylsulfanyl methane (MSM) twice daily, the toxicity and inflammation inside of the brain will be reduced. B complex vitamins, lecatin, and phosphatidyl seri will also help. With this treatment you should see improvement beginning in the first two weeks and continuing over the next two months.

Pelvic inflammatory disease

Pelvic inflammatory disease refers to chronic inflammation of the pelvic region due to ongoing infections.

Symptoms of pelvic inflammatory disease usually includes long-term inflammation and infections of the vagina, vulva, uterus, and surrounding tissues. Pain may be present for a short or long period of time and is aggravated by urination, sexual activity or yeast overgrowth. Nausea and fever may also be present.

Pelvic inflammatory disease is usually caused by bacteria, viruses, and yeast infections.

- Swallow two teaspoons of Silver Sol liquid twice a day for prevention. Drink two tablespoons twice a day for severe conditions.

- Apply Silver Sol gel topically to affected and painful area at least twice a day to destroy the pathogens that cause the pain and infection.

- To create a Silver Sol douche, mix three ounces of Silver Sol liquid with three ounces of distilled water. Pump the solution into the vaginal cavity and hold for ten minutes, then release. This should be done once a day, for five days, or until symptoms are gone.

- As an optional use, pour four ounces of Silver Sol liquid into a full tub of warm water. Soak and relax, flushing the silver water into the vaginal cavity. Twenty-five minutes is average for a muscle relaxing vaginal flush in the tub.

Personal Lubricant

Personal lubricant can be used to lubricate joints of the elbow or armpit, or anywhere skin is rubbing together and causing a rash. It is most commonly used, however, on condoms or for vaginal dryness.

By using Silver Sol gel as a personal lubricant, you will destroy bacteria, viruses, and mold—protecting both yourself and your sexual partner. It will also reduce the inflammation, swelling, and pain associated with skin rubbing against skin.

Pet Use

You can use Silver Sol liquid or gel for your pet. If a pet weighs 20 pounds, it should receive one fourth of the human dosage. In most cases, pets take one fourth to one sixth of the normal human dose, but they can safely take up to quadruple doses when they have a problem.

Pneumonia

Pneumonia is an inflammatory illness of the lung and is caused by both viruses and bacteria. The lungs can become so filled with fluid that asphyxiation occurs. Silver Sol can destroy the bacteria or the viral infection that causes pneumonia. The recommended dosage is two teaspoons, two to four times a day; 15 minutes of inhalation from a nebulizer; and intranasal spray twice a day to reduce congestion. You should expect to see benefits in the first 12 hours. In severe cases an IV protocol is an option (see also Cancer)

Post Surgical

Surgery opens the possibility of infection in wounds, stitches, and incisions. Hospital-acquired methicillin-resistant staph aureus infections (MRSA) are one of the most dangerous infections you can get. Silver Sol gel should be applied to the wound, stitches, and the surrounding area immediately after surgery. This will prevent infection, help wound healing, and reduce scarring.

Poultice

Silver gel can be placed on a body part and then wrapped in place as a poultice. This allows the wound to remain uncontaminated and to improve quicker. Silver poultice has been used in horses for years to treat infections. It can be mixed with any other desired herbs.

Prostate Disease

A prostate is the gland that closes off the flow of urine from the bladder. When the prostate relaxes, urine will flow out of the bladder and into the toilet. The prostate gland then tightens back up on the ureter and stops the urine flow. Over time, the prostrate muscle becomes bigger. If it becomes infected with bacteria, it will swell and become too large and shut off the flow of urine, making you unable to urinate.

Silver Sol can destroy the bacteria that cause the prostatitis. By drinking two teaspoons twice a day you will have enough circulating in your system to go through your urine and kill the bacteria in your bladder and prostate. Some people have felt a benefit by placing the gel between the rectum and scrotum. Using saw palmetto twice a day should also reduce inflammation in the prostate. For those who have access to a catheter, 2 oz of liquid Silver Sol can be pumped directly into the catheter and into the bladder for ten minutes where it will kill pathogens.

Psoriasis

Psoriasis is a disorder that affects the skin and joints. It commonly causes red scaly patches to appear on the skin. This condition makes you very susceptible to secondary bacterial infection getting into the cracked areas of the skin.

To fight the bacteria, apply Silver Sol gel two to four times a day, keeping skin, wounds, or rashes very moist. Drink one teaspoon of Silver Sol liquid twice daily. For very dry, scaly skin, Silver Sol liquid and gel can be mixed with Vaseline (one part gel, liquid, and Vaseline). This will keep the affected areas moisturized for a much longer period of time. Aloe vera can also be used and mixed with the gel. This will help with the most difficult situations, including Morgellon's disease.

Pus

Pus is produced when bacteria break down and destroy healthy cells. Apply Silver Sol topically to affected areas one to four times a day and drink two teaspoons of Silver Sol twice a day. If pus is being produced in your throat, e.g. sore throat or strep throat, rinse your mouth with Silver Sol liquid or apply gel to the throat. Try to keep in place for 6 minutes.

Pyorrhea (Gum Disease)

In addition to causing bad breath, gum disease erodes the gums and bones around the teeth, causing the teeth to fall out. Gum disease can be prevented by rinsing your mouth with one ounce of Silver Sol six minutes each day—the remaining rinse should be swallowed. You may also brush your teeth with Silver Sol Gel. Co-enzyme Q10 will also be of benefit.

You can expect to have a benefit after the first brushing of your teeth. After three days you will have noticeable improvement.

Rashes

Rashes can occur on any part of the body. They can come from irritation or chemicals that irritate. By putting Silver Sol gel right on the rash, you will moisturize, detoxify, and quicken healing. Apply one to four times a day and swallow one teaspoon of Silver Sol liquid twice a day.

Razor Burn

By shaving, you cut off microscopic pieces of skin, causing razor burn. Silver Sol gel can be used as shaving cream or you can wash your face with Silver Sol liquid immediately after shaving.

Shaving with acne usually results in small open wounds. In this case, you should wet your face with water, and then shave using Silver Sol gel and a razor. When you're finished, rinse off the gel and apply a thin layer of either Silver Sol liquid or gel. The wounds will improve quicker and the bacteria will die off faster. You can expect to see a benefit after the first day.

Reproductive Organs, Male

Men who have not been circumcised tend to have more hygiene problems than those who have. Uncircumcised men can apply Silver Sol gel under the foreskin to help stop fungal, bacterial, and viral infections.

> *A few years ago, AIDS was spreading very rapidly in some Southeast Asian countries. The World Health Organization did a study to find the cause. It discovered that the virus was being stored under the foreskin of uncircumcised men and then being passed to the partner during intercourse.*
>
> *To prevent the spread of disease, circumcision was made mandatory. The rate of AIDS was reduced by 95 percent in one year. Legal rulings in these countries found these mandatory circumcisions to be unlawful, and the requirement was repealed. Within three years, the number of AIDS cases was as high as it had been previously.*
>
> *Silver Sol can significantly help uncircumcised men from transmitting disease.*

Respiratory Health

Respiratory health problems are a common ailment for many of us. Colds, the flu, bronchitis, and asthma are generally caused by a virus. Silver Sol can help destroy these viruses. To prevent exposure to germs on an airplane, spray silver into your nose. Before you go to a nursery, swallow, rinse, or brush your teeth with silver gel. Use hand gel to prevent the transfer of contagious disease from hands to the face or eyes.

Germs are not the only cause of disease. An air conditioner or heater that is set too high, or on for too long, can dry out the air. This will dry out your nose, throat, and lungs. If they become chapped or cracked, viruses can enter very easily. Conversely, some homes or offices are too humid. Fungus or black mold grows in warm, moist areas including your lungs and sinuses. To avoid either of these problems, a preventative dose should be sprayed into the nose every day.

Rosacea

Rosacea is a form of bacteria that grows on the nose, making it red and swollen with pimples. This can leave very large scars. Because it is difficult to treat, doctors generally prescribe antibiotics.

Rather than use antibiotics, you can drink two teaspoons Silver Sol liquid twice a day and apply gel four times a day. Wash the nose lightly between each application. You should see a reduction of redness within the first two hours and a reduction of pimples in the first day.

Scalp Treatment

Men who shave their head can apply Silver Sol gel to the head to prevent razor burn. Placing Silver Sol gel on your scalp every night after washing will keep it moisturized and prevent it from flaking or having sun damage spots. Repeating this process twice a day will also improve the texture of your skin.

Women can use the solution to remedy hair loss caused by bacteria. Silver Sol can also help with dry scalp. Spray one to two ounces into wet hair and rub it in. Let stand for 10 minutes before rinsing.

Scars

A scar is formed when the skin is damaged and the immune system pulls it back together. The scar is made up of thickened layers of skin. Scarring can be minimized by drinking one teaspoon of Silver Sol liquid twice a day and applying Silver Sol gel directly to the wound two to four times a day. The silver will keep the wound moist and remove bacteria, mold, and viruses and help the improvement process.

Silver Sol gel can also be applied directly to scars and stretch marks, softening the skin and reducing scar size. For severe, highly-inflamed, or keloid scars, apply the gel and cover it with plastic wrap or a sterile gauze bandage.

Sinusitis

(See Nose and Sinuses)

Sitz Bath

For people who don't have the ability to get in and out of a tub, Silver Sol can be used as a spray or poured on a washcloth as a Sitz bath. By washing with a washcloth and drying with a dry towel, you can detoxify warm, moist areas that may grow yeast. It can be utilized in every orifice of the body—eyes, ears, nose, throat, mouth, vagina, and rectum.

Skin Cleanse

Cleansing the skin is very simple. Wash the skin with a mild, hypoallergenic mild soap, pat it dry and while the skin is still moist, apply Silver Sol gel. Drink one teaspoon of Silver Sol liquid twice a day for prevention.

If you have open wounds, you should apply gel more regularly. If the wound is a MRSA infection, apply Silver Sol gel every two hours to keep it moist.

According to the Surgeons Scrub Test protocol, Silver Sol gel was found to kill 99.999 percent of all pathogens, bacteria, virus, and mold for a total of four hours.

Silver Sol can also be combined with other bar or pump soaps. By heating a bar of soap and adding liquid silver, you can create a soap that has the benefits of silver. Mixing silver with pump soap gives the same benefit.

Skin Conditioner

Silver Sol makes a perfect skin conditioner because it does not contain alcohol or greasy petroleum products. To moisture skin, apply the liquid or gel after you wash your face and before applying makeup.

Skin Damage

Skin can be damaged by many things, including wind, sun, makeup, and detergent. To keep it healthy, we need a protective barrier. The protective barrier usually comes from oils that are secreted from our skin. But as we get older we secrete less and less of these protective oils. By using Silver Sol on the skin one to four times a day, the skin will stay moist and a protective anti-bacterial barrier will be created to prevent disease from entering the skin.

Skin Softening

For skin to soften, it must be moist and receive necessary nutrients. To soften skin, apply Silver Sol gel topically one to four times a day and in-gest Silver Sol liquid one teaspoon twice a day. The gel can also be mixed with aloe vera at a 1:1 ratio and applied one to four times a day.

Sore Throat

A sore throat is generally caused by bacteria, but may also be a result of a virus. To kill the bacteria that cause puss, swollen tonsils, and red spots in the back of your throat, rinse your mouth with one ounce of Silver Sol for six minutes. Allow a small amount of the solution to trickle down the back of your throat and swallow every 30 seconds. Swallow the remainder when you're done. Pump Silver Sol into your nasal cavity as needed for sore throat, congestion, or postnasal drip. Sinuses and throat need to be treated simultaneously so one does not infect the other.

My daughter is a performer who sings in front of thousands of people each night. When she travels to different cities she is exposed to cigarette smoke, pollution, and lack of sleep. These factors, combined with her singing, often result in a throat that is overworked.

To soothe her throat, we created a throat spray that consisted of a mixture of Silver Sol liquid, emollient oils, and a little bit of glycerin. After spraying it in the back of her throat, she found immediate relief. The voice box was lubricated and the Silver Sol destroyed bacteria, viruses, and mold and reduced inflammation. She was then able to sing for longer periods of time without damaging her throat.

Stomach Ache

If you have a stomachache and you don't know what is causing it, Silver Sol can usually help. By taking one ounce of Silver Sol liquid every hour for four hours, bacterial or viral infections can quickly be resolved.

Stress

Stress can be caused by any single item, even imagined worries. Silver Sol can reduce the stressful impact of bacteria, viruses, and mold on all the systems of the body. By reducing the stress, the immune system has less trouble to deal with and you will be sick less often.

Stretch Marks
(See Scars)

Stroke

Stoke is a circulatory issue that takes place inside the brain. Silver Sol liquid can help by destroying the bacteria or viruses that can cause inflammation in the circulatory system. When used after a stroke, Silver Sol can quicken the removal of blood pooled in the brain. These benefits will come by drinking two teaspoons of Silver Sol twice a day. It can also be inhaled in nebulized form.

Substance Abuse

Silver Sol gel can be applied to injection sites, abscesses, skin rashes or traumatic injuries caused by substance abuse. Swallow two teaspoons twice a day of liquid Silver Sol and apply Silver Sol gel 2-10 times a day to injured areas.

Sunburn
(See burns)

Suppository Use

The use of special Silver Sol suppositories can be very effective at delivering Silver Sol into the bloodstream. By placing a suppository into the rectum, the colon can absorb hundreds of times more Silver Sol nano-particles into the bloodstream. This phenomenon occurs because Silver Sol doesn't have to pass through acid in the stomach. Stomach acid binds with silver and serves to slow absorption. The rectal delivery of Silver Sol can be achieved by using a special Silver Sol suppository or by pushing one teaspoon of Silver Sol gel into the rectum twice a day.

Thyroid

The thyroid gland is the major gland for the hormone system of the body. Damage to this gland can result in lack of energy, too much energy, weight gain, or weight loss. Silver Sol can help because often the thyroid is damaged by a viral or bacterial infection. Drinking two teaspoons twice a day and applying Silver Sol gel to the throat will result in significant thyroid benefit.

Toenail Fungus

When Silver Sol comes in contact with toenail fungus, it will kill it within minutes. The problem is getting underneath the nail. If possible, get through the nail and clear out as much fungus as possible with a blunt instrument. The toenail fungus can then be treated by soaking the toe in Silver Sol for 30 minutes every other day.

If you can't get the Silver Sol through the nail, file down the top layer of the nail until it becomes water soluble. This will allow the silver to reach the fungus and kill it. It will take several months for the nail to grow out completely.

Tonic

Silver Sol can be used as a tonic. It helps the liver to improve itself, function better, and produce more healthy enzymes by cleaning out the bacteria, viruses, and mold. This will also result in more energy. Drink two teaspoons one to four times a day, or as needed.

Tonsillitis

Tonsillitis is the inflammation of the tonsils. It's almost always caused by bacteria. Once it begins, it often has to be resolved surgically. This is unfortunate because tonsils are a key organ in the immune system.

By rinsing with one ounce of liquid Silver Sol for six minutes each day, you will kill the bacteria. This process can be repeated daily for a very serious tonsillitis flare up. Spraying silver into the nostrils will also help. The more contact the silver has with the back of the throat, the faster it will work.

Toothache
(See cavities)

Toothpaste

Using Silver Sol as toothpaste will allow you to brush away bacteria, viruses, and mold as well as destroy bad breath. It can be mixed half and half with your regular toothpaste, if desired.

Tongue

The tongue can suffer from a number of maladies, including canker sores and bacterial and viral infections. Whatever the cause of the problem, you should rinse with one ounce of liquid Silver Sol for six minutes twice a day.

If you have a white pasty substance on your tongue, it's likely a yeast infection. You may want to brush your tongue with Silver Sol gel in addition to the rinse. For cankers, you can also apply Silver Sol gel directly to the tongue.

Tuberculosis

Tuberculosis is a common and often deadly infectious disease caused by mycobacteria. Tuberculosis has been destroyed by Silver Sol in laboratory studies. By drinking two teaspoons twice daily and inhaling from a nebulizer 30 minutes each day, you will affect the tuberculosis in both the lungs and the bloodstream.

Tuberculosis is not easy to beat. This dosage of Silver Sol may need to be followed for weeks or months. You should see benefits after the first dose and each repeated use.

Ulcers

Ulcers are caused by a bacterium called *H. pylori*. It destroys the lining of the stomach and intestines, sometimes causing a bleeding ulcer. By drinking one teaspoon of Silver Sol three to five times a day, it can enter the stomach and destroy the bacteria causing the ulcer.

It should take two weeks to get the *H. pylori* under control, but treatment should be continued for at least a month. *H. pylori* can return just by having poor hygiene, eating out at restaurants, or not washing your hands. Using Silver Sol gel can prevent its spread.

Urinary Tract Infection (UTI)

A urinary infection (UTI) is bacterial infection that affects any part of the urinary tract. The kidney, ureters and bladder are adversely affected by an invading bacteria and multiply in the urine.

The most common symptoms of a UTI are pain and burning during urination, more frequent urination, and an abnormal urgency to urinate without vaginal discharge.

UTI's are caused by bacteria, viruses and fungus that infect the genital area.

- Drink two ounces of Silver Sol liquid every hour for four hours. Since Silver Sol destroys the bacteria that causes the infection in six minutes, it is important to absorb large amounts of silver for four hours. In this way Silver Sol can wash through the kidneys and pool in the bladder. Silver Sol passes through the body unchanged so the part that pools in the bladder will still kill bacteria in the kidneys, bladder and urethra.

- Apply Silver Sol gel topically twice a day to affected area, or as needed.

- Take at least 8 billion active probiotic cultures that contain acidophilus and bifidus daily.

- Take large doses of antioxidants. This will help neutralize and clear free radicals produced by pathogens.

- Cranberry is terrific at helping reduce bladder infections.

Silver Sol can destroy bacteria that cause infections in the urinary tract in under six minutes. This means you can expect the liquid and gel to destroy the cause of the UTI as long as the Silver Sol stays in contact with the pathogen for six minutes. Most women feel noticeably better in two hours and may return to normal in as little as four to six hours.

> "I have been troubled by yeast infections and bacterial infections for twenty years. Recently I have been using Silver Sol gel twice a day on my female areas when I have sex, as a personal lubricant. I have not had a single yeast infection since using your silver gel."

Use With Other Supplements

Silver Sol reduces the burden of bacteria, viruses and yeast. As a result, supplements that help stimulate the immune system will have a greater ability to work with an immune system that has a greater capacity to perform as it should.

Vaginal Cleanse
(See Women's Issues)

Vaginal Odor

Vaginal odor can often be caused by a yeast or bacterial infection. Silver Sol can be used as a douche by pumping two ounces of Silver Sol liquid intervaginally, holding it for 12 twelve minutes, and then rinsing. Apply Silver Sol gel to a tampon and insert into the vagina.

For continued problems, Silver Sol gel can be applied to the outer areas of the vaginal opening or placed on a panty liner.

Vaginitis

Vaginitis is term used for inflammation and irritation of the vagina caused by yeast or bacteria.

Symptoms of vaginitis include redness, inflammation, itching, burning, discomfort when urinating, possibly a foul vaginal odor, and sometimes an abnormal discharge or pain during intercourse.

Vaginitis is caused by a variety of yeast of bacteria, including Candida (yeast), Gardnerella (bacteria), Streptococcus (bacteria), Herpes (virus), and Trichomonas (parasite). Candida causes a watery, white, cottage cheese-like vaginal discharge that is irritating to the vagina and surrounding skin. Bacterial causes are usually associated with a fish-like odor and are associated with itching and irritation, but not during intercourse. Viruses can cause profuse discharge with a strong fish-like odor, pain upon urination, painful intercourse, and inflammation of the external genitals.

- Drink two teaspoons of Silver Sol liquid twice a day for one week or until symptoms subside.

- You can also apply Silver Sol gel topically to affected area twice a day. Or, apply the gel to tip of a tampon and insert into vagina for 90 minutes a day so the gel can stay in contact with germs in the vagina. Do this for one week.

- To create a Silver Sol douche, mix three ounces of Silver Sol liquid with three ounces of distilled water. Pump the solution into the vaginal cavity and hold for ten minutes, then release. This should be done once a day, for five days, or until symptoms are gone.

- Take at least 8 billion active culture probiotic daily. Reduce dietary sugar and carbohydrates. And take large quantities of antioxidants daily. This will help neutralize and clear free radicals produced by pathogens.

Silver Sol can destroy bacteria, viruses, trichomonas and yeast in under ten minutes. This means you can expect the liquid and gel to destroy the cause of vaginitis as long as the Silver Sol stays in contact with the pathogen for ten minutes. The parasite trichomonas may take six weeks to eliminate. Most women feel noticeably better in one day and may return to normal in as little as two to five days.

> "I have had several infections throughout my body, including yeast and bacterial infections. I tried Silver Sol and within 36 hours the yeast infection was gone. Within another 72 hours I had my blood tested again and found it to be bacteria free. I've been taking the silver for three weeks and have not had a reoccurrence of any kind."

Varicose Veins

Varicose or "spider" veins occur in the legs (and in the rectum as hemorrhoids). It causes the blood to have difficulty returning from the feet to the heart. Veins overstretch and bloat, causing a lot of pain. If the veins rupture, it's called an ulcer. Serious problems occur if these venostasis ulcers get infected.

Silver Sol gel applied topically to the legs twice a day will help with pain and inflammation. Drinking Silver Sol liquid two teaspoons twice a day will allow the silver to circulate through the veins and arteries of the system.

Walking is essential to getting the blood flow moving again in varicose veins. I recommend stretching and walking 25 minutes each day.

Versitis
(See Arthritis)

Viral Infections
(See Anti-Viral)

Viruses

A virus is a sub-microscopic infectious agent that is unable to grow or reproduce outside a host cell. We generally fight viruses with antibiotics. However, antibiotics do not actually destroy the virus. For many viruses, such as influenza or the bird flu, there are virtually no beneficial drugs or treatment.

Silver Sol resonates at a frequency that can actually suppress and contain viral infections by interfering with the duplication and replication of viral infections. If you can stop a virus from duplicating in the first four hours of infection, you have a good chance of stopping symptoms entirely.

When the herpes virus infects the skin, we call it a canker sore or cold sore. If you use Silver Sol within the first four hours of feeling the sore, it will not even erupt. However, if you don't get it in the early phases, viral infection will duplicate and become much more difficult to control. This is why regular, preventive use is so important.

To fight viruses, Silver Sol can be taken internally as a liquid, topically as a gel, or inhaled to combat sinus problems. You can expect a noticeable benefit to be felt within the first two hours and significant benefits within the first two days.

Vitamins, Minerals, Essential Fatty Acids, Amino acids

By combining Silver Sol liquid and gel with vitamins, minerals, essential fatty acids, and amino acids, you will boost immunity by reducing stress on the immune system.

Warts

Warts are usually viral infections that have gotten under the skin and reproduced in a way that makes thickened, callused tissue around it. If you can get the Silver Sol down inside the wart it will actually kill the virus and it will die. By drinking two teaspoons of Silver Sol twice a day, it will circulate in your blood stream. Combined with topical application of the gel, you should see significant benefit.

For quicker, more complete results, pare down the wart with a sharp instrument. (Warts do not have pain receptors. When you feel pain, you've reached the skin.) Put the Silver Sol on the exposed portion of the wart.

Water Purification

Water can be purified using Silver Sol liquid. By applying four drops of Silver Sol liquid into eight-ounce glass of water, and letting it stand for about two minutes, it will purify even raw river water. Add 32 ounces of liquid Silver Sol to a 55-gallon drum of water to keep your water storage purified for years.

> *The EPA reports that 40 percent of all water is unfit to drink. I have had the experience of drinking water in foreign countries and suffering the consequences. I've gotten food poisoning twice. The first time, I did not have Silver Sol liquid and it took me two weeks to get over my diarrhea. I learned my lesson. I took silver after the second occurrence and remedied the problem within two hours.*

Wind Burn

A windburn dries out the skin. Silver Sol is very effective as a skin moisturizer. For severely chapped and bleeding skin, Silver Sol gel can be mixed with Vaseline or aloe vera, in a 1:1 ratio. This will keep the skin very moist. After one application of this mixture, Silver Sol can be applied topically on its own, as needed, for up to two weeks.

Wipes

You can create your own Silver Sol disposable wipes. Simply put Silver Sol liquid on a small napkins and carry in a zip lock bag. These antibacterial wipes can be used to clean hands, remove makeup, clean wounds, or sanitize public surfaces.

Nearly 70 percent of all contagious diseases are transferred by hand contact. These wipes will greatly reduce the amount of germs that come in contact with your system.

Women's Issues

The fact that silver is antibacterial, antiviral and antifungal makes this unique liquid the perfect vaginal cleanse. It can be very difficult to identify the source of vaginal problems/diseases due to the fact that they could be bacterial, viral or fungal. Silver Sol vaginal cleansing destroys all these sources of vaginal disease. For these and many more reasons Silver Sol can cleanse multiple sources of vaginal disease including antibiotic resistant bacteria, STDs, yeast and do so safely as a liquid or gel.

The need for improved vaginal hygiene is evident when you research the sexually transmitted diseases, yeast infections, and occurrence of viral infections that cause cancer of the uterus and cervix. Silver Sol liquid destroys the cause of numerous vaginal diseases and will become a woman's best friend when it comes to itching, cramping and yeast infections.

Wound Healing

Wounds come in many forms—burns, cuts, lacerations, bruises, broken bones. Silver Sol has been documented to help improve wound healing. In a study done at the University of Utah, pigs healed substantially faster and had less bacteria, viruses, and mold when treated with Silver Sol.

Silver Sol gel can be applied topically to any wound one to four times a day. By keeping the wound moist, it will improve quicker and with less scarring. Drinking two teaspoons of liquid Silver Sol twice a day will help improve wounds in the nose, ears, eyes, nose, throat, or any part of the body.

Yeast

Yeast can infect the vagina, cervix, uterus or vulvar opening, resulting in tissue damage of the affected areas.

Symptoms of a Candida yeast infection include redness, irritation, flaking skin, foul odor, itching, burning, and discomfort when urinating or during intercourse. May be associated with abnormal discharge. Usually causes a watery, white, cottage cheese-like vaginal discharge that is irritating to the vagina and surrounding skin.

- Drink two teaspoons of Silver Sol liquid twice a day for one week or until symptoms subside.

- You can also apply Silver Sol gel topically to affected area twice a day. Or, apply the gel to tip of a tampon and insert into vagina for 90 minutes a day so the gel can stay in contact with germs in the vagina. Do this for one week.

- To create a Silver Sol douche, mix three ounces of Silver Sol liquid with three ounces of distilled water. Pump the solution into the vaginal cavity and hold for ten minutes, then release. This should be done once a day, for five days, or until symptoms are gone.

- Take at least 8 billion active culture probiotic daily. Reduce dietary sugar and carbohydrates. And take large quantities of antioxidants daily. This will help neutralize and clear free radicals produced by pathogens.

- Capryllic acid has been shown to help reduce intestinal yeast and may help if the yeast is systemic.

Silver Sol can destroy yeast in less than ten minutes. This means you can expect the liquid and gel to destroy the cause of yeast infections as long as the Silver Sol stays in contact with the pathogen for ten minutes. Most women feel noticeably better in one day and may return to normal in as little as two to five days.

"Every time I wear nylon stockings I get a yeast infection. I have tried anti-fungal drugs, but then I get a bacterial infection. When my doctor treats my bacterial infection with antibiotics I get a yeast infection. I learned that Silver Sol destroys both yeast and bacteria. When I use it twice a day I get total control of both yeast and bacterial infections in two days."

Review: Silver Sol Gel Uses

Skin / Nails
Skin health
Healthy skin
Bites
Acne
Sunburn
Cuts/scrapes
Rashes/diaper rash
MRSA
Nail fungus
Athlete's foot
Itching
Burning
Jock itch
Yeast
Hand sanitizer
Wound management / care
Radiation burns
Chemotherapy burns
Sun burns
Cold sores / herpes shingles
First aid gel
Varicose veins
Veinous stasis ulcers
Hemorrhoids
Bruises
Healing
Mild pain
Diabetic ulcers
Bed sores
Tunneling wounds
Post surgical healing
Psoriasis
Eczema
Dry skin
Skin irritation
Antibacterial

Antiviral
Antifungal
Liver spots
Skin damage / repair
Complexion / makeup
Poison ivy / oak
Chafing
Moisturizing / flaking
Mild pain
Immune boost
Oral dental health
Sexually transmitted disease
Personal lubricant
Vaginal
Oral
Anti aging
Prevention of bacterial viruses and fungi
Dressings / band
Vaginal applications

Pathogens Destroyed by Silver Sol and the Minimum Concentration Needed (partial list)

Disease	Pathogen	Effective Concentration (Silver Sol)
Boils	Staphylococcus aureus	Killed @ 5 ppm
Osteomyelitis	Staphylococcus aureus	Killed @ 5 ppm
Bacillary Dysentary	Shigella boydii	Killed @ 2.5 ppm
Burn Infections	Pseudomonas aeruginosa	Killed @ 5 ppm
Dental Plaque	Streptococcus mutans	Killed @ 5 ppm
Diarrhea (bloody)	Shegella boydii	Killed @ 2.5 ppm
Diarrhea	Escherichia coli	Killed @ 2.5 ppm
Ear Infection	Haemophillus Influenzae	Killed @ 1.25 ppm
Ear Infection	Streptococcus pneumonie	Killed @ 2.5 ppm
Enteric Fever	Salmonella tyhimurium	Killed @ 2.5 ppm
Epiglotitis (in children)	Haemophilus influenzae	Killed @ 1.25 ppm
Eye Infections	Staphylococcus aureus	Killed @ 5 ppm
Corneal ulcers-Keratitis	Pseudomonas aeruginosa	Killed @ 5 ppm
Food Poisoning	Salmonella arisona	Killed @ 5 ppm
Food Poisoning	Samonella tyhimurium	Killed @ 2.5 ppm
Food Poisoning	Escherichia coli	Killed @ 2.5 ppm
Endocarditis	Streptococcus faecalis	Killed @ 2.5 ppm
Endocarditis	Streptococcus gordonii	Killed @ 5 ppm

Disease	Pathogen	Effective Concentration (Silver Sol)
Meningitis	Haemophillus Influenzae	Killed @ 1.25 ppm
Meninigitis	Enterobacter aerogenes	Killed @ 2.5 ppm
Meningitis	Pseudomonas aerogunisa	Killed @ 5 ppm
Meningitis	Streptococcus Pneumonie	Killed @ 2.5 ppm
Nosocomial Infections	Klebsiella Pneumoniae	Killed @ 2.5 ppm
Nosocomial Infections	Pseudomonas aeruginosa	Killed @ 5 ppm
Nosocomial Inf (Hospital)	Streptococcus pyogenes	Killed @ 1.25 ppm
Pneumonia	Staphylococcus aureus	Killed @ 5 ppm
Pneumonia	Haemophilus influenzae	Killed @ 1.25 ppm
Pneumonia	Pseudomonas aeruginosa	Killed @ 5 ppm
Pneumonia	Streptococcus pneumonie	Killed @ 2.5 ppm
Respiratory tract infection	Streptococcus pyogenes	Killed @ 1.25 ppm
Respiratory tract infection	E. coli	Killed @ 2.5 ppm
Respiratory tract infection	Klebsiella pneumoniae	Killed @ 2.5 ppm
Scarlet fever	Streptococcus pyogenes	Killed @ 1.25 ppm
Septicmia	Enterobacter	Killed @ 2.5 ppm
Sinus Infections	Haemophilus influenzae	Killed @ 1.25 ppm

Disease	Pathogen	Effective Concentration (Silver Sol)
	Streptococcus pneumonie	Killed @ 2.5 ppm
Impetigo	Staphylococcus aureus	Killed @ 1.25 ppm
Skin Infections	Staphylococcus aureus	Killed @ 5 ppm
Skin Infections	Streptococcus pyogenes	Killed @ 1.25 ppm
Strep Throat	Streptococcus pyogenes	Killed @ 1.25 ppm
Suppurative Arthritis	Haemophilus influenzae	Killed @ 1.25 ppm
Throat Infections	Haemophillus influenzae	Killed @ 1.25 ppm
Tooth Decay	Streptococcus mutans	Killed @ 5 ppm
Urethritis (men)	Trichomonas vaginalis	Killed @ 10 ppm
UrinaryTract Infections	E. coli	Killed @ 2.5 ppm
UrinaryTract Infections	Klebsiella pneumoniae	Killed @ 2.5 ppm
UrinaryTract Infections	Pseudomonas aeruginosa	Killed @ 5 ppm
UrinaryTract wInfections	Streptococcus faecalis	Killed @ 2.5 ppm
Vaginitis (women)	Trichonomas vaginalis	Killed @ 10 ppm
Wound Infections	Escherichia coli	Killed @ 2.5 ppm
Wound infections	Enterobacter aerpyogenes	Killed @ 2.5 ppm
Wound Infections	Klebsiella pneumoniae	Killed @ 2.5 ppm

Disease	Pathogen	Effective Concentration (Silver Sol)
Wound Infectons	Pseudomonas aeroginosa	Killed@ 5 ppm
Wound Infections	Streptococcus faecalis	Killed @ 2.5 ppm
Yeast Infections	Candida albicans	Killed @ 10 ppm

INDEX

A

Abscesses 44
Aches 44
Acid Reflux 45
Acne 46
Age Spots 47
Aging 48
Air Toxins 33
Allergies 49
Alzheimer's Disease 49
Amino acids 134
Anti-Aging 49
Anti-Bacterial 50
Antibiotic Alternative 53
Antibiotics and Silver 47
Anti-Fungal 50
Anti-Tumor 51
Anti-Viral 52
Appetite Suppressant 53
Arthritis 54
Asthma 54
Athlete's Foot 54
Attention Deficit Disorder 47
Autism 55

B

Backache 55
Bacteria 19, 56
Bacterial 99
Bacterial Infections 56
Bad Breath 56
Bedsores 57
Bio-Terrorism 9
Black Mold 57
Bladder Infection 57

Blood Cleanser 58
Body Odor 58
Boils 59
Bones 59
Bowels 60
Brain Cleansing 60
Breast Cancer 60
Bronchitis 61
Bruises 61
Bug Bites 62
Burns 62

C

Cancer 63
Candida 67
Canker Sores 66
Cardiovascular Disease 67
Carpal Tunnel Syndrome 67
Cataracts 67
Cavities 68
Chafing 68
Chicken Pox 70
Children 69
Cholesterol 69
Chronic Fatigue Syndrome 71
Circulation 71
Circulatory System 42
Cleanse 34
Cleansing 71
Colds 72
Colitis 72
Colon 72
Compress 73
Congestion 73
Conjunctivitis (Pink Eye) 74
Constipation 73
Contagious Diseases 8

Coughs and Croup 74
Crohn's Disease 74
Cuticles 75
Cysts 75

D

Dandruff 75
Dengue Fever 76
Depression 76
Dermal Renewal 76
Detox Bath 77
Diabetes 77
Diaper Rash 78
Diarrhea and Dysentery 78
Digestive 43
Digestive System 78
Diverticulitis 72
Diverticulitis and Diverticulosis 79
Dry Skin 79

E

Ear Drops 79
Ear Infections 79
Endometriosis 80
Enema 81
Energy 82
Epidemic 6
Epidemics 82
Epilepsy and Seizures 82, 83, 84
Epstein-Barr Virus 83
Essential Fatty Acids 134
Eye Lift 84
Eyes 84

F

Face Lift 85
Facial Mask 85
Facial Peel 85
Facial Treatment 85
Family Use 86

Fatigue 86
Fertility 86
Fevers 87
Fibromyalgia 87
Fingers 87
Flu 89
Follicle Detox 88
Food Poisoning 88
Foot Bath 88
Foot Odor 89
Fungus 20

G

Gallbladder Disease 90, 91, 92
Gargle 91
Gastritis and Gas 91
Genital Herpes 91
Gingivitis 92
Gum Disease 121

H

Hand Disinfectant 92
Hand Restoration 92
Hay Fever 92
Headaches 93
Healing Gel 93
Heart Disease 94
Hemorrhoids 93
Hepatitis 94
Herpes 95
High Blood Pressure 95
Household Disinfectant 96
Human Papilloma Virus (HPV) 96
Hypertension 97

I

Immune Modulator 98
Impetigo 98, 99
Infections 99
Infectious Disease 99

Inflammation and Swelling 100
Influenza 100
Inhaled Silver Sol 100
Intestinal Detox 100
Intravenous Treatment (IV) 100
Irritable Bowel Syndrome 72, 100
Itching and Scaling 101

J

Jock Itch 101
Joints 101

K

Keratosis 102
Kidney Disease 102

L

Lacerations 102
Leichmaniasis 105
Leprosy 104
Leukemia 104
Lip Balm 105
Lips 105
Liver Disease 105
Lung Disease 106
Lupus 106
Lymphatics 108

M

Makeup Base 109, 112
Makeup Irritation 109
Malaria 108
Male 122
Memory Enhancement 110
Menopause 110
Migraine Headaches 110
Minerals 134

Mold 20
Mold and Fungus 111
Mononucleosis 111
Mouth Wash 111
Multiple Sclerosis 113
Myocardial Infarction 114

N

Neck Firming Cream 114
Nerves 114
Night Cream 114
Nose and Sinuses 115
Nose Drops 115

O

Obesity 115
Orifices 116
Osteoporosis 116

P

Pain 116
Pancreas 116
Pandemics 82
Parasites 117
Parkinson's Disease 117
Personal Lubricant 118
Pet Use 119
Pneumonia 119
Post Surgical 119
Poultice 119
Prostate Disease 120
Psoriasis 120
Pus 120
Pyorrhea (Gum Disease) 121

R

Rashes 121

Razor Burn 121
Reproductive Organs 122
Reproductive System 42
Respiratory Health 122
Rosacea 123

S

Scalp Treatment 123
Scars 123
Seizures 83
Sinusitis 124
Sitz Bath 124
Skin Cleanse 124
Skin Conditioner 124
Skin Damage 125
Skin Softening 125
Sore Throat 125
Stomach Ache 126
Stress 126
STRESS 34
Stretch Marks 126
Stroke 126, 127
Sunburn 127

T

Thyroid 127
Toenail Fungus 127
Tongue 129
Tonic 128
Tonsillitis 128
Toothache 128
Toothpaste 129
Tuberculosis 129

U

Ulcers 129, 130, 131

V

Vaginal Cleanse 131
Vaginal Odor 131, 132
Varicose Veins 133
Versitis 133
Viral 99
Viral Infections 133
Viruses 20, 134
Vitamins 134

W

Warts 134
Water Purification 135
Water Toxins 32
Wind Burn 135
Wipes 136
Women's Issues 136
Wound Healing 136

Y

Yeast 137, 139